The International Library of Psychology

AN INTRODUCTION TO INDIVIDUAL PSYCHOLOGY

Founded by C. K. Ogden

The International Library of Psychology

INDIVIDUAL DIFFERENCES
In 21 Volumes

I	The Practice and Theory of Individual Psychology	*Adler*
II	The Neurotic Constitution	*Adler*
III	Duality	*Bradley*
IV	Problems of Personality	*Campbell et al*
V	An Introduction to Individual Psychology	*Dreikurs*
VI	The Psychology of Alfred Adler and the Development of the Child	*Ganz*
VII	Personality	*Gordon*
VIII	The Art of Interrogation	*Hamilton*
IX	Appraising Personality	*Harrower*
X	Physique and Character	*Kretschmer*
XI	The Psychology of Men of Genius	*Kretschmer*
XII	Handreading	*Laffan*
XIII	On Shame and the Search for Identity	*Lynd*
XIV	A B C of Adler's Psychology	*Mairet*
XV	Alfred Adler: Problems of Neurosis	*Mairet*
XVI	Principles of Experimental Psychology	*Piéron*
XVII	The Psychology of Character	*Roback*
XVIII	The Hands of Children	*Spier*
XIX	The Nature of Intelligence	*Thurstone*
XX	Alfred Adler: The Pattern of Life	*Wolfe*
XXI	The Psychology of Intelligence and Will	*Wyatt*

AN INTRODUCTION TO INDIVIDUAL PSYCHOLOGY

RUDOLF DREIKURS

Foreword by Alfred Adler

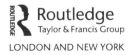

LONDON AND NEW YORK

First published in 1935 by
Kegan Paul, Trench, Trubner & Co., Ltd.

Published in 2001 by
Routledge
2 Park Square, Milton Park, Abingdon, Oxfordshire OX14 4RN
711 Third Avenue, New York, NY 10017

First issued in paperback 2014

Routledge is an imprint of the Taylor and Francis Group, an informa business

© 1935 Rudolf Dreikus
Translated from the German by Edna G Fenning

All rights reserved. No part of this book may be reprinted or reproduced
or utilized in any form or by any electronic, mechanical, or other means,
now known or hereafter invented, including photocopying
and recording, or in any information storage or retrieval system, without
permission in writing from the publishers.

The publishers have made every effort to contact authors/copyright holders
of the works reprinted in the *International Library of Psychology*.
This has not been possible in every case, however, and we would
welcome correspondence from those individuals/companies
we have been unable to trace.

British Library Cataloguing in Publication Data
A CIP catalogue record for this book
is available from the British Library

An Introduction to Individual Psychology
ISBN 978-0415-21055-3
Individual Differences: 21 Volumes
ISBN 0415-21130-1
The International Library of Psychology: 204 Volumes
ISBN 0415-19132-7

ISBN 978-1-138-87537-1 (pbk)
ISBN 978-0-415-21055-3 (hbk)

CONTENTS

	PAGE
FOREWORD (by Alfred Adler) . . .	vii
COMMUNITY FEELING	1
FINALITY	11
THE SPOILT CHILD	18
SNUBBING	23
THE INFERIORITY FEELING AND STRIVING FOR SIGNIFICANCE	25
ORGAN INFERIORITY	34
HEREDITY AND EQUIPMENT . . .	43
THE FAMILY CONSTELLATION . . .	47
THE LIFE PLAN AND THE LIFE STYLE . .	55
THE FICTIVE GOALS — THE MASCULINE PROTEST	60
CONSCIOUSNESS AND CONSCIENCE . . .	65
THE UNITY OF THE PERSONALITY . . .	72
NEUROSIS	77
CRIME AND INSANITY	89
UPBRINGING	95
PSYCHOTHERAPY	112
THE THREE LIFE TASKS—WORK, LOVE, FRIENDSHIP	120
EPILOGUE	147

[v]

FOREWORD

By

ALFRED ADLER

IT must be about twenty years since I tried to foretell the future of Individual Psychology in some such words as these. Individual Psychology, which is essentially a child of this age, will have a permanent influence on the thought, poetry and dreams of humanity. It will attract many enlightened disciples, and many more who will hardly know the names of its pioneers. It will be understood by some, but the number of those who misunderstand it will be greater. It will have many adherents, and still more enemies. Because of its simplicity many will think it too easy, whereas those who know it will recognize how difficult it is. It will bring its followers neither wealth nor position, but they will have the satisfaction of learning from their opponents' mistakes. It will draw a dividing line between those who use their knowledge for the purpose of establishing an ideal community, and those who do not. It will give its followers such keenness of vision that no corner

FOREWORD

of the human soul will be hidden from them and it will ensure that this hard-earned capacity shall be placed in the service of human progress.

The author of this book is well fitted to speak in the name of Individual Psychology. His life, his work, his first book on *Psychic Impotence* (published by S. Hirzel, Leipzig) are all evidences of a mode of thought which is characterized by acceptance of Individual Psychology, enthusiasm for co-operation and specialized knowledge. It may well be that the introduction of his new book will disclose to many darkened minds the secrets after which they are groping.

An Introduction to Individual Psychology

THE COMMUNITY FEELING

WHAT forms the character of a human being? What makes a man act as he does? What forces govern all the activities of the human mind? These are the fundamental questions which psychology tries to answer. So many people are now exploring them and there are so many theories that we are apt to feel confused. Some people assume that the life of each individual is determined by the experiences and desires of his ancestors (Jung). Others regard the Psyche as the battlefield of the most various instincts, corresponding to various forms of the sexual instinct (The Psycho-Analysis of Freud). Many think that the most complicated behaviour patterns are the outcome of the automatic action of certain reflex mechanisms, which are built up and maintained by habit (The Reflexology of Bechterev) Others look upon man with all his functions as the mere product of his environment, which through the medium of education directs his behaviour (The Behaviourism of Watson). A number of other theories have been advanced by different pioneers in order to explain psychic phenomena. The leading idea of the Individual Psychology of Alfred Adler is found in

[1]

COMMUNITY FEELING

his recognition of the importance of human society, not only for the development of individual character, but also for the orientation of every single action and emotion in the life of a human being.

There are certain species that cannot exist without close contact with their kind. Man belongs to these. Nature has not fitted him to fight singlehanded. He is not equipped in the same way as other animals for the struggle for existence. He neither has weapons of attack in the form of sharp teeth, great physical strength and powerful claws, nor is he able to defend his life by extraordinary swiftness or inconspicuous smallness. It seems that men formed herds exactly like other herding animals simply because this was necessary in order to preserve existence.[1]

Most of us have no adequate idea of the extent to which man nowadays depends on co-operation with his fellow men. We have only to think of the thousands of people whose labour we employ each day, or need only consider how many people have co-operated to provide our houses, clothing, food, and a thousand other necessities of our daily lives.

---

[1] It is a well-known fact that birds fitted to share the struggle for existence and to rear their young in pairs, gather together in flocks before undertaking the difficult task which a long journey involves. Likewise weak, defenceless animals form herds in order to organize a better defence. The formation of a community is a very effective way of preserving existence, and therefore it is often adopted, but it is not the only way. Animals similar to those living in communities are also frequently found leading a solitary mode of existence.

COMMUNITY FEELING

For centuries man has lived in more or less close social relations with his fellow men and has adapted himself to a system of division of labour and mutual assistance. During infancy the human child is one of the most defenceless creatures in the world. He cannot find his food without help, nor even walk alone. In exercising all his functions he depends on the co-operation of others.

The question now arises : *to what extent* can living in a closely knit community form the character of an individual ? It might seem, as the Psycho-Analysis of Freud maintains, that human instincts adapt themselves only incompletely and faultily to the reality of close social relationships, and that the human Psyche is indeed at the mercy of incompatible demands—the need for adjustment to the community, and the needs of innate instincts. Nevertheless, observation shows that not only among men, but also among animals, close social relationships, with the very delicate adjustment to the claims of others which is involved in such relationships, decisively affect the nature and characteristics of species, and even enable some individuals to revolt against laws of nature which otherwise prove generally irresistible. All living creatures feel a compulsion to maintain life, which causes them to seek for food, and a desire to propagate themselves, which finds its fulfilment in love. And yet under certain circumstances men refuse to obey their natural instincts. Children

[3]

COMMUNITY FEELING

may choose to starve themselves if they think such tactics are the best they can adopt in a struggle with their parents. Prisoners starve themselves as a form of protest. Thousands upon thousands of people who wish to evade the claims of a love relationship suppress every sexual emotion. Man has tamed his natural instincts and subordinated them to his attitude to his environment, and we find that the bees go to even greater lengths. They have reduced the sexual instinct—otherwise an all-powerful instinct, dominating the whole sphere of nature—to a precisely ordered function, which they regulate in accordance with the needs of their commonwealth at any given moment. They not only command means enabling them to decide arbitrarily whether they will produce males or females, but they can also allot the sexual function to certain individuals and later deprive them of it. Thus even creatures like bees, who live in the most closely knit communities known to us, can reverse generally valid biological laws. This supports Alfred Adler's view of the importance of society for the development of individual character among human beings.

When we observe people we find that the nature, character and actions of an individual are determined by the experiences he encounters in the community within which he grows up. Here we seem to approach Watson's theory of Behaviourism, according to which man is the mere product of

[4]

COMMUNITY FEELING

his environment. But if we look deeper we find that in addition to the influence of environment another vitally important circumstance remains to be considered. Different people respond in different ways to the same experiences and influences. Man does not merely react. He adopts an individual attitude. The attitude adopted depends on the impressions the individual forms in early childhood. Environment is indeed a determining factor. Yet this environment is not the individual's real environment, but merely his environment as it appears subjectively to him. Therefore the decisive factor for the development of character is not the influence of environment, but the attitude to environment which the individual takes up. Man develops his characteristic behaviour—his character—solely by opposition or support, negation or affirmation, acceptance or non-acceptance.

Man's urge to adapt himself to the arbitrary conditions of his environment is expressed by the community feeling innate in every human being. Its roots go centuries deep. But this innate social characteristic, which is common to all, must be developed if the individual is to be qualified to fulfil the complicated demands of the community in which the civilized adult lives.

The human community sets three tasks for every individual. They are : work, which means doing useful work, friendship, which embraces social relationships with comrades and relatives, and love,

[5]

COMMUNITY FEELING

which is the most intimate union with some one of the other sex and represents the strongest emotional relationship which can exist between two human beings.

These three tasks embrace the whole of human life with all its desires and activities. All human suffering originates from the difficulties which complicate the tasks. The possibility of fulfilling them does not depend on the individual's talents nor on his intelligence. Men of outstanding capacity fail where others with far inferior powers achieve relative successes. It all depends on community feeling. The better this is developed and the happier the relationship between the individual and the human community, the more successfully does he fulfil the three life tasks, and the better balanced his character and nature appear.

The community feeling is expressed subjectively in the consciousness of having something in common with other people and of being one of them. People can develop their capacity for co-operation only if they feel that in spite of all external dissimilarities they are not fundamentally different from other people. A man's ability to co-operate may therefore be regarded as a measure of the development of his community feeling.

A specific example will help us to visualize the situation more clearly : A man becomes a member of a group, a club, a political party or some other association. His community feeling expresses

COMMUNITY FEELING

itself subjectively in his consciousness of membership. Expressed objectively it will show how far he is able to co-operate in life. On his community feeling depends how soon he makes contact with others, whether and to what extent he can adapt himself to others, whether he is capable of entering into other people's feelings and of understanding other people. A man who thinks only of himself, of how he is to uphold his own dignity and of the part he means to play, is sure to cause trouble within his circle of friends and acquaintances.

Readiness to co-operate, which is one of the characteristics of a good comrade, is tested most rigorously in difficult situations. Most people are perfectly willing to co-operate so long as everything is to their liking. It is much more difficult to remain a good comrade in an uncongenial situation. If the tie which binds a man to a community is weak, he will easily break away as soon as anything he does not like happens. The stronger his feeling of membership, the more surely will he remain loyal to the community, even when he cannot enforce his own wishes. We never find conditions which entirely conform to our wishes in any human relationship, be it friendship, the family, love or work. Sooner or later, therefore, we are bound to become involved in critical situations, and the way we behave then will show whether we are community minded or not.

Another characteristic of the good comrade is his

[7]

COMMUNITY FEELING

readiness to demand less than he offers. Nowadays most people brought up in large towns are spoilt children, who measure their happiness and satisfaction only by what they get. This is a grave error, for which thousands pay in unhappiness and suffering. People who make it their object to get as much as possible are always clutching emptiness. They are insatiable. Only a rare and brief moment of attainment rewards months or years of covetousness and ambition. None but those who can seek their happiness as a part of the whole, that is to say, in the contribution they themselves can make to the community, can feel satisfied with themselves and their lives. The community feeling therefore is expressed by willingness to contribute without thought of reward.

We shall have a sufficiently reliable criterion as to whether any given action takes into account the needs of the community, if we observe to what extent the action is objective. Objective action implies suitable and right behaviour in any situation. It is impossible to prescribe how anyone should behave in this or that situation. Every situation involves a special and very complicated set of circumstances, and no one can say beforehand how they should be handled. The crucial questions are :—Have the rules of community life been mastered ? Is the individual ready to subordinate himself to them ? If so, he will know more or less the right course to adopt in any situation, no matter

[8]

COMMUNITY FEELING

how difficult, because he will be able to regard his problems objectively. He will never be baffled if he can subordinate ego-centric wishes to the objective needs of the community.

In spite of the apparent chaos of present-day social relationships we have rules to guide us. These rules are clear to everyone even though they have never been definitely formulated. Each person becomes aware of the relentless logic of life as soon as he tries to escape it. Success or failure is the answer given by the community to fulfilment or non-fulfilment of the life tasks.

Frequently a man whose contacts with the community are superficial appears to be consistently successful, while another who always seemed to have adapted himself sufficiently to the needs of the community may suddenly break down. The explanation is that the strength of the community feeling is not always put to the proof. If a man is spared by favourable circumstances from undergoing rigorous tests, he may easily give others the impression of being able to solve every problem. He is like a pupil who for some time escapes examinations. His knowledge is taken for granted. If a man has to endure great hardships his lack of training for life will be revealed more quickly. But sooner or later everyone has to show how far his community feeling has developed. This moment decides whether his life can be happy or not. Therefore disaster and misfortune are not inevitable

COMMUNITY FEELING

causes of suffering and discouragement, but test situations, which prove whether people are ready to co-operate. While one accepts defeat, another keeps a brave heart. He never loses his feeling of comradeship with other people and in the end he wins through.

Yet the community feeling does not mean, as misrepresentations of the teachings of Alfred Adler often incorrectly state, simply a feeling of belonging to a certain group or class of people, or benevolence towards the whole race. Sometimes the interests of various groups conflict. (This is the dilemma of a workman on strike, who may hesitate between his family's welfare and the need for solidarity with his fellow workers.) In such perplexing situations the community feeling causes us to see that the interests of the super-ordinate group, which are justified on the ground of objective needs, have the first claim on us. We certainly want to do what we can to help men to found a community embracing the whole human race, to whose interests all the special interests of individuals and groups would be subordinated. But in practice we are still a long way from realizing this ideal. The community feeling has no fixed objective. Much more truly may it be said to create an attitude to life, a desire to co-operate with others in some way and to master the situations of life. Community feeling is the expression of our capacity for give and take.

[10]

FINALITY

CLEARLY the attitude adopted by the individual to the problems of community life could not determine the development of his character were he driven from the beginning in a certain direction by inherited tendencies. If instincts and other innate forces governed his behaviour at every juncture, only a certain adaptation and modification of his personalty in response to the conditions of his environment would be possible. It is found, however, that all the characteristics of the individual, and indeed his whole personality, are developed by the attitude he adopts to his environment in early childhood. Actually the personality is developed in this way only if human soul-life is teleologically orientated. In other words, the object which the individual pursues in his actions is the decisive factor. We must admit this if we believe that his attitude to his environment consistently determines all his actions, and the sum of his actions—his personality.

But are we justified in rejecting causality, the law which was hitherto thought to determine the mental development of all human beings, in favour of the view of finality, which prefers to stress the fact that the individual can select from a great

[11]

FINALITY

variety of ways and means ? We now find that quite apart from psychology, science in general is becoming concerned to an ever increasing degree with this much debated problem—causality or finality.

Probably the Neo-Vitalists were the first to assume that the question of use was the decisive law governing all forms of life. They reached their assumption after studying the evolution of species and organs, and above all the biological processes of the body. In their view all symptoms of illness and all pathological changes are not effects produced by some harmful agent, but weapons for defeating it. The classical example of this is inflammation, the " purpose " of which is to destroy the invading bacteria by multiplying leucocytes. Similarly every biological change is understood solely in the light of the purpose it is intended to accomplish.

Quite apart from such biological trains of thought, Alfred Adler stresses the fact that all living things move, and that every movement must have a goal. So, according to Alder, all living things seek a goal. With regard to man in particular, Alfred Adler declares that it is impossible for us to understand his behaviour and actions unless we know their goal.

This teleological mode of thought, which appears to contradict all our accustomed beliefs, formerly met with the keenest opposition from science, and

[12]

FINALITY

was frequently rejected as unscientific. The last great development of the natural sciences in particular was based on acceptance of the doctrine of causality, which regards every occurrence as the simple effect of a certain cause. The theory that a connection other than that between cause and effect may be at the root of any observed occurrence is extremely difficult to grasp, yet Individual Psychologists are now experiencing the great satisfaction of seeing it accepted by what is surely one of the exactest sciences, Physics. Although this repudiation of the law of causality made it possible to ascertain the boundaries of causality only in the realm of the smallest atom, it involved such a fundamental change in the laws of thought that the violence and frequency of the debates on the subject among students of physics are understandable. This overthrow of causality in another field at the same moment is an apparent coincidence, but has many parallels in the history of the development of human thought, and there can be no doubt that it contributed to the great advance made in the field of psychological research.

When an individual acts in a certain way we naturally ask why he does so. This indeed was the only question asked by psychology before Alfred Adler. In the early days of psychological research people tried to find a purely mechanical and material explanation for all actions. They believed that impressions were transmitted to the

[13]

FINALITY

body through the sense organs, and then indirectly — through a reflex or brain process — a certain action was liberated. Freud was the first to discard the theory that human actions are governed by physical laws, and emphasized the need for the acceptance and recognition of purely spiritual laws for man, but even he was misled by the principle of causality, and looked to the past for the explanation of all human actions. He declared that all former psychic experiences were reserves of certain psychic energies, and therefore must be recognized as compulsive factors, which necessarily produce a certain result.

The principle of causality, whether it was handled by materialists or by Freudians, was never particularly useful or practical. The subtler the methods employed by the former in tracing the springs of man's actions, the more chaotic was the picture in which they sought to reproduce multitudinous sense irritations and reflex channels, and to prove that man is governed by purely physical laws. On the other hand, as a result of Freud's attempt to find a law of energy embodying his discovery that man was dominated by a psychic force, rash theories were advanced. These theories could never be verified in practical life. They could only be demonstrated in the special atmosphere of a psycho-analyst's consulting room. The next step was to discover an entirely different law of movement for human beings.

[14]

FINALITY

Adler made a remarkable discovery when he found the motive force of every human action in the goal of the action. This discovery is fully confirmed by personal experience, as far as the normal life of a healthy human being is concerned. Objections could only be raised with regard to some human actions which appear to be useless and senseless and to be performed against the agent's wish, or at least without his wish. Far from rousing opposition, however, Adler's views as to the purposive quality of even these aberrations are supported by the observations of almost all famous psychiatrists, including some who otherwise have very little to say in favour of Individual Psychology, such as Wagner-Jauregg, Bonhöffer, Kahn, etc. It is true that they go only a little way in accepting the teleological law. They do not recognize the importance of the tendency betrayed at the beginning of apparently unwilled actions except in connection with outbreaks of hysteria and neurosis which follow accidents. But if they make only these exceptions, they admit by implication that even when a man does not consciously recognize the fact that his actions have a certain goal—even when he feels that he performs them against his own will—his actions may still have a goal.

The phenomenon of the unconfessed goal is closely connected with the problem of consciousness, which requires a more detailed discussion

FINALITY

than it can receive in this chapter. Here we will limit ourselves to observing that it may not be very obvious to an ordinary man that all his actions have a goal ; so that a situation in which he feels as if he is being driven first one way and then another by conflicting wishes, and is not clear as to what he really wants, may give him the impression that the human mind is the battlefield of various instincts and impulses, and that the resulting action is to be attributed to the victory of the strongest instinct. Nevertheless, since we regard the human being as an undivided personality, we judge not only the resulting action, but also the previous hesitation as a consistent and reasonable " action," serving its particular purpose as effectively as a simple unfettered expression of will may serve a different purpose. This subject will be discussed at greater length in the chapter on the unity of the personality.

It is obvious from everything that a human being does that he has the power to orientate towards a certain environment, for ultimately his action and inaction are decided solely by the question of " which way ? " He is not driven through life by his past, but impelled to go forward into the future —and the force that impels him is not an external force. He moves of his own accord. All his actions, emotions, qualities and characteristics serve the same purpose. They show him trying to adapt himself to the community. Character is not

[16]

FINALITY

determined causally by equipment or instincts. Neither is it formed by environment, which would bring us back once more to causal determination. Belief in finality is based on belief in the " creative power," which enables a man to seek his goal as he judges best. Man acts far more than he reacts. At this point Individual Psychology comes into contact with the views of Bergson, who recognizes the essential indetermination of every living substance in his theory of the " élan vital."

THE SPOILT CHILD

FROM the very first day of his life the human child has a place in a community with which he has to make contact in order that the necessities of his life may be satisfied. His first way of communicating with his surroundings is by screaming. He cries for his mother to come when he feels hungry or experiences any discomfort, and no matter how small the infant, his screaming is regulated according to the parents' behaviour.

From the very outset the infant has certain social functions to perform. This makes some kind of discipline essential. The infant's first task is feeding. It is comparatively easy to train a healthy child to perform this task, that is to say, to teach him to co-operate satisfactorily with the mother. Every child will, of course, offer some resistance to the first attempt to fix regular feeding hours. He will scream at other times, but if the parents are sensible and patient, they will not allow this to deter them from enforcing their system. The child will soon give up screaming, and within a few days will automatically accustom himself to regular feeding hours and even exhibit a certain degree of satisfaction in keeping them. So for the first time in his life he adapts himself and

[18]

THE SPOILT CHILD

co-operates with others as a member of the community.

Unfortunately at this early stage serious mistakes are very frequently made. From motives of false pity over-anxious parents try to " spare the poor little thing " in every possible way. " Oh, he'll accustom himself to regular hours later on when he's stronger." It is very natural for the parents of a child who is delicate or ill to feel extremely concerned. By the doctor's advice possibly even these parents will attempt to teach a child regular habits, but if the child has some difficulty in learning to suck, and regularly loses strength during the first days of his life, they will not have the heart to " let him go hungry " when he cries to be fed. The result is that discipline is disregarded.

The older the child grows the more difficult it becomes to teach him disciplined habits. Each day strengthens his resistance to any change from irregular hours, once he has grown accustomed to them. At the same time the steady development of his lung powers becomes more and more patent. Then, as irregular hours prevent him from thriving the mother's anxiety increases. But the more she tries to establish an orderly régime, the more the child screams, and after a shorter or longer period of hesitation the mother gives way. The child thus makes his first important discovery—that he can get his own way by screaming, or at least

[19]

THE SPOILT CHILD

make his mother take him up and rock him in her arms or give him something to pacify him. (Freudians make the fatal mistake of regarding the child and the whole of mankind as obedient to the " pleasure principle ", so that every frustration must be the counterpart of a " pleasure ideal ". They forget that this applies only to people who have not become happy members of the community. Pleasure may be derived even from discipline, if it appears reasonable, and after all, pleasure simply expresses acceptance).

The result of the various forms of spoiling and pampering is that the child grows up in a hot-house atmosphere and enjoys artificial privileges, which exempt him from the natural discipline of community life. He need not submit to the rules which apply to all the other members of the first community he encounters in life—the family. Special precautions prevent him from knowing any discomforts. Artificial warmth envelops him. He need not earn recognition by any achievements of his own. Pity and indulgence shield him from all the disagreeable consequences of his actions. He never learns to put up with anything he does not like. Somebody is always ready to help him and spare him the necessity of making any effort. Over great anxiety holds him back from encountering dangers which spell risk and demand courage.

Parents who spoil a child make it very difficult for the child to become a useful member of the

[20]

THE SPOILT CHILD

community. Most of us are spoilt children. This is not the less true because many of us do not feel at all as though we had ever been spoiled. For every attempt to spare the child the necessity of submitting to discipline must result in the child's disliking discipline, in his adopting a hostile attitude towards it, and ever afterwards resenting even the modicum of discipline which has to be maintained wherever people live in a community. (In this connection Freud speaks incorrectly of the "destruction of instinct" which civilization inevitably involves.)

Whenever a child is spoilt a time always comes when at last an attempt is made to discipline him. The child naturally resists this. He cannot see why something which he was hitherto allowed to do should suddenly be forbidden once and for all. He does not feel that order is a wise law, enabling people to live together in a community, but a mere parental whim. Frequently, therefore, all that sticks in the memory of spoilt children is the struggle with the parents, who for their part generally make use of highly unsuitable methods to achieve by force an object that could have been realized without any difficulty at all, if they had previously shown less weakness.

The only safe rule for ascertaining how much spoiling a child has had and the degree of hostility to discipline this has engendered is provided by asking to what extent the child is aware of being

[21]

THE SPOILT CHILD

spoiled. A child is particularly alive to the situation if, being the only child in the family, he alone is pampered and allowed to dictate to the other members of the family and regulate their lives, as if they existed merely to minister to his wants. He will not regard his pampered childhood in the same light if later on he has to live in very uncongenial surroundings. This alone shows that the child himself is fully responsible for the meaning he attaches to the parents' behaviour, and for the attitude to his past which he adopts in consequence.

SNUBBING

SOONER or later the spoilt child feels frustrated and realizes that a right which he believes he is justified in claiming is being curtailed. Spoiling actually amounts to disregard of the child's right to become independent and to learn at an early age what the requirements of life are. Usually spoiling is far less the result of consideration for the child, as the parents assert, than of consideration for their own feelings, because they cannot bear seeing the child wear out his strength, suffer in any way or get into difficulties. Doting parents deprive the child of other vital rights. These are the parents who cannot allow a young child to sleep regular and sufficient hours, merely because they want to dandle him, or because visitors coming to the house want to admire him. The desire to parade a child in front of visitors encroaches on his right to play with other children. Excessive anxiety deprives him of his right to freedom of movement.

The child is frustrated and deprived of his rights in a particularly flagrant manner if the parents interfere with discipline and make disturbances from no motives of love for the child, but solely out of regard for their own interests. If excessive love often makes it difficult for the child to become

SNUBBING

a happy and useful member of the community, as much may certainly be said of unkindness, which denies that the child has a place of his own in the family. Children whose parents hate them because they came into the world unwanted are often denied their rights in a very shameful way. Sometimes parents turn away from a child because she is a girl instead of the boy they had been hoping to have, or because they see a certain resemblance between the child and some one they dislike. Sometimes a parent has a spite against a stepchild. The parents' unkindness is always felt more keenly by the child if he is very much indulged by another person, who probably acts from some motive of compensating justice.

Snubbing always arouses resistance. Often the child's resistance or obstinacy may appear to have been destroyed by beatings or by other measures of force adopted by his elders. But under cover of even the most abject submissiveness the child will still achieve his object—retreat from the community, evasion of all the implications of communal life. Such is the effect produced on the child if he thinks he is only hated. Not infrequently the child misjudges the parents' behaviour. He may believe that they care little for him, even when this belief is not justified in reality. On the other hand the child will not want to retreat into himself if he fails to observe that his parents really hate him, and remains unaware of being snubbed.

[24]

THE INFERIORITY FEELING AND STRIVING FOR SIGNIFICANCE

WE have seen how both spoiling and snubbing may hinder the child from becoming a useful member of the community. We must now discover what factor comes into play in the mind of the spoilt child and the snubbed child alike. How can experiences so different from each other as spoiling or snubbing have the same effect—that of disturbing the community feeling innate in every human being ?

When we examine this paradox more closely we find that whether the child is spoilt or snubbed, he always develops a feeling of his own relative inferiority, which causes him to resist the rules of the community and to adopt a hostile attitude to the community. The behaviour of all children and all adults establishes the general validity of the following law : The natural community feeling of every human being reaches its limits when feelings of inferiority arise.

A diagram may make the situation easier to grasp.

The individual tries to get himself accepted by the community (C). He therefore moves along the line a—b, that is to say, if no obstacle checked his advance towards the community he would move

INFERIORITY FEELING

along this straight line towards C. Man would only act and develop in response to the conditions of his community. The force ruling his actions and psychic life would be undisturbed community feeling.

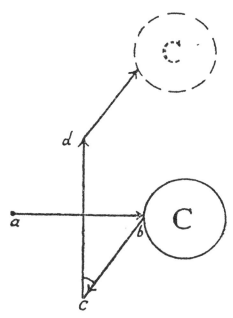

But we have seen that difficulties may prevent the child from becoming a happy and useful member of the community. He imagines that the community is a hostile world and feels unable to cope with it. It seems to him that the community repulses him and tries to force him down (in the direction shown by the line b—c in our diagram).

In the minds of children, and later also of adults,

STRIVING FOR SIGNIFICANCE

all ideas of being repulsed are inevitably connected with the subjective feeling of being " less " than other people. It is immaterial whether the child accepts the superiority of others as a result of spoiling, because he underestimates his own strength and regards his dependence on the superior strength of others as something to be taken for granted, or whether as the result of snubbing he has come to believe that the superior power of others will always be victorious. Invariably the child imagines that the contrast between his power and the power of other people means that the other people are " worth more " than he is.

The child resents this feeling of being low down in the scale, and very soon all his actions show that he is moving in a new direction. In response to his innate community feeling he persists in trying to get himself accepted at any cost by the community. But as he assumes that his value is too small or his strength inadequate, he thinks that he can reach the community only by first climbing to a higher position. Consequently, as already stated, he moves in an entirely new direction, shown in our diagram by the line c—d. Any person who labours under a sense of inferiority always tries to obtain power of some kind in order to cancel the supposed superiority of other people. His feeling of inferiority impels him to strive for significance.

It should always be remembered that the inferior-

INFERIORITY FEELING

ity feeling is a subjective feeling. The inferiority may exist only in the imagination of the individual when he compares himself with others. The inferiority feeling is in a very deep sense quite independent of a man's true value, because when he compares himself with other people he gives them fictive values. Anyone who doubts his own value always over-estimates the capacities of other people. Therefore neither the absence nor the presence of inferiority feelings is any index to a man's real value. Some extremely valuable and successful people suffer acutely from inferiority feelings. On the other hand we may not be able to find a trace of an inferiority feeling in a lunatic. An individual's estimates of his own value, which find expression in inferiority feelings, are based entirely on his personal attitude to the community and to other people. That is to say, they are founded on his own opinions. He plays the rôle of both prosecutor and judge at his own trial. The low value he assigns to himself often appears to be connected with actual failures, but there can be no doubt that anyone who believes that his failures prove his lack of value deceives himself. Very frequently people come to entirely wrong conclusions about their own successes or failures. Often a man disparages everything valuable that he has done, and attaches far too much importance to a completely senseless failure. In the end all failures turn out to be not so much the causes of

STRIVING FOR SIGNIFICANCE

inferiority feelings as inevitable consequences of such feelings. As surely as people expect little of themselves they meet with failures.

People betray their inferiority feelings and their consequent desire for significance in an endless variety of ways. Wherever we observe human mistakes and faults (which we only regard as mistakes and faults because they violate the rules which enable people to live in a community), we shall always find a feeling of inferiority causing the individual to renounce the direct line of approach to the community. Every fault, whether it is a defect of character, or a single instance of mistaken conduct, grows out of evasion of some social task. People evade social tasks in order to conceal their own deficiencies and to avert a dreaded failure.

There are two chief modes of evasion. On the one hand people may run away from their opportunities, avoid making decisions, limit their sphere of action and try to gain time or set a distance between themselves and other people. We all take out several of these " insurance policies " during our lives. Our object is to conceal a feeling of inferiority either from others or from ourselves. On the other hand, people may try to deflect the line they take in an upward direction. They try to gain special significance by achievements in some particular field. If they can do so by means of useful achievements they will perhaps appear

[29]

INFERIORITY FEELING

to be perfectly capable of adapting themselves to the community, although their deepest impulses were fear of the community and a tendency to retreat. Sometimes, indeed, fear is the incentive for outstanding achievements, which contribute to human progress and the development of culture. It is only when a man does not seek success in the form of useful achievement, or undervalues contributions he can make to the community because his need for personal significance is too great, that he acts in response to his will-to-power without regard for anything useful and wastes his strength " on the useless side of life." He despises his fellow-men, his environment and life itself, and sets his heart on achieving meretricious successes at any price, even at the price of his own suffering. The martyr's rôle of suffering is a particularly clear example of the way in which a man appears to reverse real circumstances in a struggle with a powerful régime, since the helpless martyr triumphs over the brute force of those who are actually more powerful than he.

Disparagement of others and of life itself may be expressed in a number of ways. Sometimes it is displayed openly in dissatisfaction with everything, or extremely cutting criticisms. Equally often it poses as goodwill towards men. Extravagant idealism or exaggerated moral tenets and ethical principles set up such high standards for other people that they necessarily appear small

[30]

STRIVING FOR SIGNIFICANCE

and worthless. Disparagement of reality is also expressed in fantasy and melancholy, and most frequently in daydreams, which relegate every-day-life and the present moment entirely to the background.

These capacities for taking cover and finding a fictive increase of power receive their training in childhood. A spoilt child in particular quickly succeeds in converting his feeling of inferiority into a strong desire for significance. It is easy enough for him to play a special rôle, since he enjoys importance by the mere fact of his existence, even though he has no useful achievement to his credit. He is most afraid of not being noticed, because he thinks this means he is no longer important. He claims every minute of his mother's attention. He tries to stop her talking to grown-ups and other children, and insists on her sitting with him while he is going to sleep. But if he feels that he has not sufficiently safeguarded his weak position, or believes that it is being threatened in some way, he adopts stronger measures. He behaves naughtily, retreats into shyness, refuses to eat and gets into tempers or panics. In brief, he employs all the tricks of a cunning little animal in order to make the grown-ups do what he wants them to do. The spoilt child with an inferiority feeling always tries to tyrannize in some way over other people, especially if he happens to be an only child or the youngest of a family.

[31]

INFERIORITY FEELING

So spoilt children develop various characteristics, by means of which they try to overcome their feeling that they have no value for other people. The deficiency or supposed deficiency they feel most keenly is their most vulnerable spot. Often they are timid because they magnify dangers and consequently try to give them a wide berth. A child who feels that his own strength is inadequate grows to need support. He tries to make other people his slaves ; he lacks firmness of character ; he becomes unruly and easily gets tired, with the result that the grown-ups themselves have to carry out his tasks if only for the sake of peace and quietness. Instead of finding happiness in successful achievements, he looks for cheaper sources of satisfaction ; he becomes frivolous, idle, and pleasure-seeking, and escapes into fantasies and daydreams.

A child who gets the impression that people neglect and hate him tries to revenge himself for his feeling of helpless frustration by giving them as much trouble as he can. There is nothing very attractive about the headstrong, grimy child who knows just how to touch the grown-ups in their weak spots and, of course, uses his knowledge to protest against their treatment of him. He behaves wilfully at school and becomes generally unpopular with his teachers. His fondness for giving the grown-ups unpleasant shocks may even encourage him to develop criminal tendencies,

[32]

STRIVING FOR SIGNIFICANCE

for a perverse wish to be disagreeable is a common motive for lying and stealing.

It would be necessary to quote individual case histories in order to prove that all faulty behaviour in childhood and adult life alike is the result of unsuccessful attempts to overcome feelings of inferiority in misguided ways. Yet we know that the inferiority feeling is a driving force which produces the most various travesties of asocial conduct, because all impulses directed against the community vanish in proportion as the inferiority feeling diminishes and the individual learns to estimate his own value more correctly. Once a human being declares war on the community, peace cannot be restored until he has found a correct standard of values.

ORGAN INFERIORITY

ORGAN inferiority affords a particularly plain example of the part played by inferiority feelings and the way they may develop or be overcome. Any organ or organ system in the human body may be affected by an organ inferiority.

By organ inferiority is meant not an absolute defect but a relative weakness of an organ as compared with the functions of other organs, so that subjectively the individual experiences difficulty in exercising his functions. Now, since the use of functions constitutes the child's principal task in the community, anything which seems to make it harder to regulate his functions also gives him the impression of being worth less than other people—that is to say, gives him a feeling of inferiority. Some examples will probably make this clearer.

An organ inferiority which affects the alimentary tract does not in the least mean that the digestive organs are unhealthy. It is true, however, that if a child is delicate all the functions of the digestive organs are more laboriously regulated and more easily disturbed than they are in a healthy child. It is more difficult to get the delicate child to eat

[34]

ORGAN INFERIORITY

regular meals and he easily falls into irregular ways with regard to defecation. He therefore finds it more difficult to be an orderly member of the community and to acquire habits of cleanliness. All the child's difficulties confirm his belief that it is too hard for him to regulate the functions of the digestive organs, though the other people who are older have no difficulties of any kind.

All physical disturbances in the exercise of functions can operate as organ inferiorities. A child with eye trouble may grow up inattentive. An inferiority of the uro-genital organs may lead to difficulties in the control of the bladder function. An extremely delicate constitution, which curtails the length of time that can be spent in physical exertions, or stoutness accompanied by ungainliness and clumsiness are resented and rated as organ inferiorities. Similarly a child may resent being unusually small—in fact, anything which gives him the impression that he is of less value physically than other people.

Relative unskilfulness of the right hand in a child who is born left-handed may also have the effect of an organ inferiority. When this child tries to learn to shake hands in the ordinary everyday way with the right hand, he will experience considerable difficulty. He will then be inclined to exaggerate his incapacity for learning to do things correctly.

At this juncture a vital question presents itself

[35]

ORGAN INFERIORITY

for consideration :—What is the outcome of organ inferiority or what response does it evoke ? There are two diametrically opposed ways of dealing with this as with all other situations involving psychological difficulties. The decision is simply a question of more or less courage. Does the child allow the difficulties resulting from an organ inferiority to discourage him or not ? On this depends the course he subsequently takes. An organ inferiority is never static. It is not something that merely exists. Rather it operates dynamically through the final use to which it is put.

Let us consider in more detail the very common organ inferiority of constitutional lefthandedness. The child experiences difficulty in using his right hand. The grown-ups find fault with him and scold him. The child gradually loses faith in himself and becomes careless and clumsy. When he has to learn to write he writes badly. Nobody realises that because he has been lefthanded from birth he naturally finds it difficult to use his right hand. He is always being reminded of his extraordinary carelessness and clumsiness. If owing to excessive spoiling the child has lost faith in his own capacities at a very early age, he will regard every difficulty which crops up as insurmountable and give up trying to acquire manual dexterity because he is clumsy with his right hand.

Among children who have become extremely discouraged the organ inferiority of the right hand

[36]

ORGAN INFERIORITY

may easily produce permanent defects in the exercise of important functions. These children will always be clumsy. Their handwriting will be bad. They will have hard work in making up their minds to perform manual tasks and consequently they will tend to become slovenly. As a result of being lefthanded (a peculiarity which is not always very evident) a child may even have difficulty in learning to read. So difficulties viewed in a spirit of growing discouragement produce various defects.

The child may respond in this spirit to organ inferiorities of the alimentary tract or of the bladder. Great difficulty is experienced in regulating the functions of the digestive organs and the child develops dirty habits. If he is severely punished he will become bad-tempered. If his parents show anxiety he will take advantage of his difficulties to get more attention. In short, the child will retreat further and further from a courageous solution of his difficulties, and his feeling of inferiority will grow in proportion.

But this is not the only way of responding to an organ inferiority. If the child has not become discouraged he treats his difficulty very differently. He observes it and tries to overcome it. He pounces most eagerly on his greatest difficulties and tries to excel chiefly in activities in which these difficulties seem calculated to hamper him. He wants to master his difficulties and the requirements of life at the same time. And success is within his

[37]

ORGAN INFERIORITY

reach. Such a child later accomplishes outstanding achievements in the very field where he at first encountered difficulties. The early clumsiness of lefthanded children gives place to special dexterity, which, as often as not, finds expression in artistic productions. Children with organ inferiorities of the alimentary tract persevere in their efforts to gain control and mastery of these functions until they become extremely fastidious and methodical. Frequently a special value attached both to eating and defecation replaces the original difficulties.

These responses to difficulties all confirm a fundamental law for overcoming inferiority feelings, which was already stated by implication in the previous chapter.[1] Whenever an attempt is made to compensate for an inferiority feeling, this is never done by way of actual compensation, but always in the sense of overcompensation.

The reason for this is clear. If anyone makes great efforts so as not to be worth less than others in a certain field he lives in constant dread lest he should find that he is, and that other people will know it also. And even when he has already become as expert as other average people, he will still be afraid lest there should be someone who excels him. So he is continually drawn towards the goal of perfection, which is never attainable in practice.

Everyone who, instead of being discouraged,

[1] Pages 27 and 29.

ORGAN INFERIORITY

tries to overcome organ inferiorities, obeys this law of overcompensation. Very musical people are often found in families where defects of hearing are remarkably common, and artistic people in families with all kinds of defects of eyesight. So we begin to understand a fact which at first seems very perplexing—namely, that geniuses, artists and great men often exhibit unmistakable signs of organ inferiority in the very field of their outstanding achievements. Examples of famous musicians whose hearing was impaired by constitutional organ inferiorities like Franz and Smetana, famous orators whose speech organs were affected by certain weaknesses in early life like Demosthenes and Viktor Adler, famous painters with defective eyesight like Manet and Lenbach, and famous writers who combined a romantic imagination with defects of eyesight like Karl May and Jules Verne, can be multiplied at will and clearly prove that frequently an organ inferiority provides the incentive for artistic achievements. It is by no means the only incentive for undertaking the special training which necessarily precedes any outstanding achievement. No doubt there are many reasons why a child endeavours to achieve a special success in a special field ; yet constitutional organ inferiority provides a stimulus which, far from being rare, is extremely common.

The presence of a constitutional organ inferiority cannot, however, be deduced from its consequences,

[39]

ORGAN INFERIORITY

that is to say, from defects or from overcompensation. It is justifiable to speak of an organ inferiority only when it has been sufficiently proved that there was a constitutional defect which rendered the exercise of a function difficult. Proof is furnished chiefly by the family anamnesia, i.e., when organic disorders of a certain organ system occur extremely frequently among the nearest relatives. Suspicion that an organ inferiority exists may be confirmed by a number of other indications, such as birthmarks, the development of feverish skin disorders in that part of the body which is nearest to the organ thought to be affected by an inferiority, or by subsequent organic deterioration of the organ ; for instance, by the appearance of tumours, or by otosclerosis when organ inferiority of the ear is suspected. There are several signs that betray latent lefthandedness— as for example, a steady preference for using the left hand for performing small unimportant actions, like clapping, cutting cards, etc.

On the other hand, we should not, of course, hold an organ inferiority responsible for every difficulty encountered in the use of a certain organ. It is indeed true that as a human being develops, any disturbances in the normal performance of functions are most likely, *ceteris paribus*, to make common cause with an organ inferiority. That is why disturbances of functions are so often used to reinforce resistance or become modes of evasion.

[40]

ORGAN INFERIORITY

A child can just as well use his organs (as, for example, his digestive organs) to promote a disturbance, even when they are entirely free from organ inferiorities. The only safe guide is to see whether by these means he achieves his object, that is to say, whether other people and, above all, his parents, submit to the disturbance. Any healthy organ can be trained to promote a disturbance ; and under some circumstances even a secondary functional disturbance, for which the way has been prepared by sufficient training, may later lead to relative overcompensation. For example, children who hungerstrike without the stimulus of organic defects may later attach importance to eating plentiful meals.

This human tendency to overcompensate for inferiority feelings plays a most important part in the history of mankind. Just as an organ inferiority may lead to the performance of outstanding artistic achievements in a particular field, so every endeavour to rise higher, and every achievement which promotes the development of the race and advances civilization, is the outcome of the wish to ease a gnawing feeling of inferiority. All human beings experience moments of anxiety or at least are troubled on account of the insufficiency of the body, which is felt like an organ inferiority. For the human body is not only little fitted to endure the material hardships of life. It is also subject to illness and death. Man knows the

ORGAN INFERIORITY

cosmic laws of origin and dissolution. He perceives his own smallness in the universe and is aware of the anguish which is inherent in everything that lives. Besides, as children we have all felt small and inferior as compared with the grown-ups, and we are all impelled to overcome difficulties. Extreme physical defencelessness not only apparently caused men, as already noticed, to form communities, but also led to the development of the human intellect. In compensation for inadequate physical strength, man acquired the capacity for using powerful forces outside his own person, such as stones, weapons, animals, the forces of nature and machinery.

In the life of an individual also the feeling of inferiority may become the incentive for achievements which, while they help him to go forward and develop more fully, also promote the advance and higher development of the whole race. The inferiority feeling ends in retreat and self-frustration only when the individual has become so discouraged that he no longer relies on achievements " on the useful side of life."

[42]

HEREDITY AND EQUIPMENT

THE observations concerning the importance of organ inferiority in general and the implications of overcompensation in particular which Alfred Adler made when he began his investigations formed the foundation on which the whole structure of Individual Psychology was later erected, and at the same time provided an entirely new standard for rating the importance of hereditary equipment.

Laws of heredity come into force wherever life is handed down from generation to generation and there can be no doubt that they are applicable in a very real sense to human beings. Man has from birth many natural propensities, capacities and weaknesses like any other animal, but he is fundamentally different from all other animals in that the part played in his development by a community life gives him a mastery over his " natural equipment " such as has never hitherto been observed even among animals living in the closest of communities.

The previous chapter dealt with the technique of this mastery. Let us now look more closely at the question of equipment.

It is obvious that if a certain function of the body falls into disuse it becomes increasingly difficult to

[43]

HEREDITY AND EQUIPMENT

exercise it. Any capacity may go to waste for want of training in childhood. The most valuable talent—amounting even to capacity for outstanding artistic achievements—is useless to a child who neglects and indeed probably refuses to train it out of spite against his parents. The same applies to a gift for mathematics or manual dexterity—in fact, to any capacity for achievement in any field. All human methods of achievement are extremely complicated and cannot be mastered without training. If training is neglected abilities remain undeveloped. It is not even enough to have a special talent.

Thus it becomes clear that what determines the way in which the personality finally develops is " not the equipment we bring with us, but the use we make of it."[1] By the interplay of neglect and training each individual forms his capacities and qualities as his individual position within the community demands. He is free from the restrictions of causal determinism as represented by his equipment.

Therefore what a man has become is in no way indicative of the quality of the equipment he had at the outset. In every individual we see only the phenotype, from which we can deduce little about the genotype. With man we cannot as with other animals learn much from the study of a series of generations, not only because the series we are able

[1] Alfred Adler.

[44]

HEREDITY AND EQUIPMENT

to observe are generally too short, but also because in every separate case the significance of psychological phenomena can be understood only through a course of psychological analysis which covers a limited space of time, that is to say, only by observing what is going on at the present moment, and not by looking back to ancestors.

Scientific investigators find it easier to deal with man's physical inheritance. But it is necessary to be cautious in discussing even this subject, as processes which appear to be purely physical may be changed in individual cases by psychological factors. In most accounts of the connection between physical structure and character the physical factor generally, though not always, takes precedence. Character and physical structure do indeed affect each other in turn, but a man's psychic personality, just as much as his innate capacities and the physical conditions of his life, represents material for him to utilize when choosing his personal objective.

Man also exercises choice in his response to the so-called " instincts," which appear to govern him like all living creatures. These are primarily the instinct for self-preservation expressed by hunger, and the instinct for continuing the race, expressed by love. These inborn urges appear to dominate all animals with the exception of those living in very close communities, like ants, bees, men and their domestic animals. Among these, as has

HEREDITY AND EQUIPMENT

already been shown, numerous examples may be observed of complete control gained over the urges of hunger and love. So long as these and other instincts are amenable to reason we have no ground for assuming that our actions are arbitrarily determined by our instincts. Only when our actions are contrary to common sense do we appear to have any argument for the alleged supremacy of " instincts."

Upon closer examination, however, unreasonable behaviour usually proves to be the outcome of hostility to the order established by the human community. In themselves hunger and sexuality are forces without direction. The individual personality alone sets a goal before the " instincts " and gives them a special content. Hunger then becomes appetite and sexuality becomes love. All the complications and conflicts involved in the " satisfaction of the instincts " arise in this way. The complications are not indications of the strength of the " instincts " but give expression to individual proneness to create problems. Hunger allows comparatively little scope for the attainment of personal motives—thirst practically none. Hence they can be more easily satisfied. But many personal objectives may be concealed beneath love and other instinctive emotions.

THE FAMILY CONSTELLATION

THE theory that each person has an innate individuality from birth appears to find confirmation in the fact that children in the same family are different from each other. It is indeed admitted by those who uphold this theory that the parents' behaviour can influence the child's attitude, and through this the development of his character, but they say that the parents treat all the children alike and that therefore the differences between the children must be attributed to their equipment.

Upon closer examination, however, it is found that each child has an essentially different position in the family and must see all the circumstances of his childhood in an entirely different light. Besides, in practice the parents never treat two children alike, but behave very differently to each. There may be a difference in the affection they feel for the children, and there certainly will be in the opinions they hold about them. At this point it might be useful to suggest briefly some points of view which are characteristic of the different children in a family.

Let us begin with the eldest child. The outstanding fact of his childhood is that at first,

[47]

THE FAMILY CONSTELLATION

though only for a limited period, he was the only child. While he is the only child he is likely to get far too much spoiling. He is the centre of attraction and the special object of his parents' care. Then he suddenly finds himself in the thick of a tremendous experience. A brother or sister is thrust upon him. Even if the first child is already a few years old he is hardly ever able to gauge the situation correctly. He notices only that another child now continually monopolizes his parents, especially his mother, who devotes herself to him, and lavishes any amount of time and care on him. He readily believes that the newcomer will rob him of her love. He cannot know, of course, that he was once looked after by his mother in exactly the same way and that all the care she bestows on the second child does not mean that she loves him more. So, feeling that he has been set aside, the eldest child frequently shows understandable jealousy when another child is born, even if before the birth of this child he longed for a brother or sister

If the mother can make the elder child aware of his undiminished value by pointing out to him his importance as the elder and therefore more advanced child, and so enlist his will to co-operate, he will adapt himself to the new situation with comparative ease. But the parents may not understand what is going on in the elder child's mind and may grow impatient over his unfounded

[48]

THE FAMILY CONSTELLATION

jealousies and ailments. If, as is most probable, they then take the younger child under their protection in order to defend him against the elder child's overbearing conduct, the elder child may easily give up trying to win good opinions by making himself useful, as he probably could do, but become obstinate and try to take up his parents' attention by resorting to every possible trick that naughtiness can suggest to him.

Even if under the most favourable circumstances two children of the same parents manage to live together in apparent harmony they may become involved in a rivalry which, though not always openly declared is none the less deadly. The elder child tries either to preserve his superiority or, if it is already endangered at least to prevent the younger child from attaining superiority. The older the second child becomes and the greater the part he takes in activities which formerly appeared to be the prerogative of the elder child, the more reasonable seems the latter's fear of being overtaken and surpassed. He endeavours in every way to safeguard his superior position as the elder and more advanced child.

What has been said about the first child suggests the situation which the second child meets. He never loses sight of the brother or sister who has got a short start of him. He fully realizes that the elder child is endeavouring to impose his superiority on him. He resents the imputation that he is less

[49]

THE FAMILY CONSTELLATION

important. He regards everything the other child can do and he himself cannot do as an indication of his own inferiority. So every second child tries to catch up to the first child. This explains why second children are generally much more active than first children, whether they choose the line of useful achievement or naughtiness.

The outcome of the rivalry between the first and second child depends mainly on the help each child gets from others. The one who has the parents on his side is, of course, in a stronger position. Occasionally also an elder child, like Esau in the Bible, may renounce his birthright because he simply gives up trying to hold his position against the attacks of the younger child. The child who emerges victorious from the struggle is more likely to be successful throughout the remainder of life than the other, who will always accept defeat too easily. The duel between the two first children generally decides the whole subsequent course of their lives.

As frequently observed, however, one child is not always victorious in everything and the other defeated in everything. One achieves superiority in one province and the other in another. When this happens we have the plainest proof that the development of individual character is determined even in the smallest detail by the attitude to environment adopted in childhood.

It is not too much to say that we usually find a

[50]

THE FAMILY CONSTELLATION

fundamental difference both as regards nature and character between the first two children. This becomes easy to understand if we remember that each of the two tries to achieve superiority in the very field where the other encounters difficulties. The younger child in particular develops an almost uncanny power for detecting the elder child's weak points and proceeds to win praise from parents and teachers by achieving brilliant successes where the other has failed. When there is keen rivalry and only a slight disparity of ages between two children of the same parents, we often find that later on at school each does particularly well in subjects in which the other does badly. If one child is puny and ailing the other grows up robust and hardy. If one is exceptionally clever at lessons the other tries to win recognition by success in something else. A child whose rival is very attractive in appearance will probably try to impress people with his intelligence or courage ; but obviously it would be impossible to enumerate all the variations produced by this preference for antithesis.

The antithesis often seems to be based on inherited capacities, especially if each of the children appears to take after a different parent. But a child's psychological attitude can make the physical likeness to one parent more pronounced. A certain similarity may result from imitation of this parent's facial expressions, gestures, attitudes and peculiarities of speech ; for a characteristic

THE FAMILY CONSTELLATION

cast of features is gradually formed by constant repetition of the same facial movements.

To a far greater extent, however, similarity of nature and character is the outcome of the child's special training. It is true that we cannot tell beforehand why the child should imitate this particular parent. We can only be wise after the event. Often the child tries to acquire the characteristics of the parent whose ally in family quarrels he has become. He seizes on these characteristics because he hopes to reach the goal of superiority by evincing like the parent who is his ally a definite character as against the other members of the family. Actuated by the same desire to gain power, many children imitate the parent with whom they are in direct conflict.

Freud fully recognizes the importance of this situation for the formation of a child's character. But while in his eyes it is indicative of a very complicated development of the Ego-ideal, which makes the feared and hated parent a secret object of love, Individual Psychology has a very simple explanation to offer. The parent who counters many wishes and is very severe is the child's conception of power. This explains why children imitate the parent they fear. They merely wish to have this parent's power. So we are able to formulate the only fundamental law governing the development of the child's character : *he trains those qualities by which he hopes to achieve independ-*

[52]

THE FAMILY CONSTELLATION

ence or even a degree of power and superiority in the family constellation.

In a large family of children the conflict between the first and second child is repeated under some form or other lower down in the family, but it generally tends to be less fierce. Consequently children who come in the middle of a family usually develop more balanced characters. The third child frequently sides with one of the two elder children. Often two children lower down in the family treat each other as rivals like the first and second children.

The youngest child has a special rôle to play. Not merely one child, but all the other children are ahead of him. All the other members of the family spoil him and regard him as the little one. He generally develops characteristics which make it likely that other people will help him to shape his life, such as helplessness, a winning nature and whimsicality. But youngest children often prove very clever if their smallness becomes an impulse for outstanding achievements.

A boy in a family of girls and vice-versa one girl in a family of boys is in a special position. These children will form a characteristic appreciation of their rôles and will develop qualities which help them to play these rôles. They often over-estimate the importance of the rôle of their own sex, because this represents the essential difference between themselves and all the other children.

[53]

THE FAMILY CONSTELLATION

Naturally the importance they attach to the rôle played by their own sex also depends on the value attached to it within the whole family and above all on the value attached by the parents to their own sex rôles, with the possible superiority of either the father or the mother.

So it becomes understandable why people adopt a certain attitude to their fellow beings in childhood, and why above all they get a definite idea of themselves. We must now try to see why a line of conduct which was reasonable and understandable in childhood is pursued throughout the rest of life.

THE LIFE PLAN AND THE LIFE STYLE

AT birth the child encounters an unknown world and a mode of life which he has to learn. Above all he has to learn the rules of the human community, to perform functions and master the tasks set by life. At first the child sees only that part of life and of the human community which is bounded by his environment, the family in which he is living. To him this environment means " life " and the members of the family seem to be " the human community " and he attempts to adapt himself to them.

He seeks to maintain himself within this concrete community by means of a variety of acquired accomplishments, characteristics, modes of behaviour, capacities and artifices. The difficulties he encounters have been outlined in previous chapters. If we now examine the situation more closely we find that the child is bound to get the impression that the difficulties he personally experiences are the absolute difficulties of life. He does not realize that the other people round about him are involved in conflicts of an entirely different nature. His growing intelligence prompts him to overcome the difficulties of his position, so far as this appears possible, unaided and alone.

[55]

THE LIFE PLAN

This explains why every individual by the time he is four to six years old has developed a definite character and why any fundamental change of character after the fourth to sixth year is hardly possible. Character is therefore simply the manifestation of a certain plan which the child has evolved and to which he will adhere throughout the rest of his life.

A child's life plan does not grow out of a certain peculiarity nor out of isolated experiences, but out of the constant repetition of certain difficulties, real or ˙imagined, which he encounters. Each individual will find out special ways and means which appear to be serviceable for his special plan. Out of the individual's special life plan develops the life style which characterizes him and everything he does. His thoughts, actions and wishes seize upon definite symbols and conform to definite patterns. The life style is comparable to a characteristic refrain in a piece of music. It brings the rhythm of recurrence into our lives. Everyone offers the stoutest opposition to any attempt that is made for whatever reason to change his life style.

So we can understand why an only child becomes timid if he feels that to be alone and unaided is the greatest hardship in life—a difficulty which cannot be surmounted, and why he betrays himself at every turn if he rates his importance in the community in terms of the recognition and consideration

[56]

THE LIFE STYLE

he gets. We can understand why the eldest child of a family may live in constant dread of being supplanted and why a second child may always feel at a disadvantage. It also becomes clearer why in later life these people continue to behave as though they were still living in the same situation as in childhood.

In addition to the difficulties encountered within the family circle, the child's social environment plays an important part in fixing the life plan. The family's position in the community may cause the child to conclude that community life involves certain social and economic dangers. Social conditions may determine the ideas he forms about his position in relation to his comrades and playmates—in short, in relation to all his fellow beings. In order to contend with all these dangers he tries to evolve a definite plan.

An imaginary example may make the situation plainer. Let us picture a child growing up in a colony of thieves. He learns that if he is to maintain himself at all he must keep a careful watch on his property, distrust others and defend himself against their depredatory tendencies. Later on he is able to leave the colony and live in the ordinary world where thieves do not compose the entire population. But he continues to behave as before, because his chief fear in life is to become the victim of a thief. He does not believe the assurances other people give him that this fear is

[57]

THE LIFE PLAN

excessive, and is always looking out for incidents which appear to justify his behaviour. Whenever anything is stolen he feels triumphant. If on the other hand he hears of an honest finder who has given up his find, he is inclined to dismiss the report as untrue and say that he is not simpleton enough to believe such a fantastic story. And if sooner or later it becomes impossible for him to doubt a person's honesty, he gets out of his dilemma in another way. This man, he says, must certainly be crazy—at least, he is different from normal people.

Probably, however, his companions will appeal to his better nature and tell him that he really must give up his unreasonable mistrust. He may then try to prove that he is broadminded and actually give his confidence to some person ; but it is practically certain that the first person he trusts will turn out a thief—partly because people of this type have been familiar to him from childhood and he feels secretly at home with them, and partly because he can turn the incident to account as an irrefutable argument : " There now, you see what happens if I believe what you say ! " After this he can continue to practise without let or hindrance the rules of conduct he learnt as a child and hold the wickedness of other people responsible for all the disagreeable experiences he goes through in consequence.

This obviously imaginary example of a single

THE LIFE STYLE

peculiar circumstance exaggerated out of all proportion to the real conditions of life illustrates firstly the importance of the life plan. Secondly it shows that it is possible to persist in the course first chosen only by grossly misrepresenting facts encountered later. We are forced to regard everything we see and all our experiences from a biased standpoint if we wish to preserve intact the mistaken ideas about life and ourselves which we formed as children. The private brand of logic which each person evolves appears to justify his mistaken behaviour, and prevents him from seeing that most of the difficulties and disappointments in his life are the logical consequences of mistakes in his life plan.

THE FICTIVE GOALS—
THE MASCULINE PROTEST[1]

As we have seen, what most often endangers the success of the individual's attempts to fit into the community and his hope of living a sane and happy life is the feeling of his own inferiority. So each human being's chief problem is the problem of his own value. As long as his value remains unchallenged he is in no danger of creating problems for himself—not even when he encounters external difficulties which do not involve psychological problems but most often provide a stimulus for consistent effort.

Uncertain people who come into sharp conflict with their surroundings, including neurotics of all kinds, have the greatest difficulty in solving this problem of their own value. But no human being is entirely free from neurosis, least of all the modern city dweller, since the first human community he knew was most probably the disintegrating family of the present day.

In obedience to the human law of overcompensation, every human being's life is directed towards the goal of increased personal importance. As the

[1] In this decisively important chapter I have reproduced many of Alfred Adler's own statements and quoted largely from his writings.

[60]

THE MASCULINE PROTEST

individual, while remaining unconscious that he has set this goal before himself, nevertheless gives a bias to his whole life and to all his actions in his endeavour to reach it, this fictive goal is the key to the riddle of his whole personality. The stronger his feeling of inferiority the more complicated his behaviour becomes.

The child who has a constitutional inferiority—we may include the ugly child, the pampered child and the child who has been brought up too strictly in the same group—will make great efforts to escape the many hardships of his life and to ward off the danger of a defeat which seems to threaten at some distant future date. He feels that he needs a landmark to keep in view because he has no sense of direction. So he has recourse to a helpful fiction. He regards himself as unskilful, inferior, subordinated and uncertain in judgment. He finds a guiding line which becomes the normal line followed by his thoughts and actions when he takes as his second fixed point his father or mother, whom he endows in imagination with all the power in the world. He then tries to rise above his uncertainty to the supposed security of his all-powerful father, and even surpass him.

All feelings of uncertainty and inferiority give rise to a need for an objective to guide, reassure and make life bearable. The result is the crystallization and hardening of every characteristic which represents a guiding line in the chaos of life and so lessens

[61]

THE FICTIVE GOALS

uncertainty. In the many complications and perplexities of life the guiding lines are intended to divide right from wrong and above from below.

In the eyes of the child brought up in the modern civilized world the concepts masculine and feminine are just such a pair of contraries corresponding to above and below. Our civilization is mainly a masculine civilization, and the child gets the impression that while all adults enjoy superior powers the man's position is superior to the woman's. Although she occasionally manages to encroach on his privileges, he still appears to be more powerful, more important and more fortunate. He has greater physical strength ; he has the advantage in height ; he has a more powerful voice. As soon as the child is able to appreciate the numerous social privileges enjoyed by men he may easily come to regard the male as the symbol of power. His concept of masculine will include whatever is " above " and his concept of feminine whatever is " below ". The woman's rôle seems to be one of service and longsuffering. The boy's goal of superiority prompts the resolve : " I'm going to be a real man." From this standpoint he protests against any treatment which seems likely to lower his value. So the " masculine protest " may become the main fiction of his whole personality.

We find that women also have masculine goals if they are unwilling to accept their sex rôle. Some

[62]

THE MASCULINE PROTEST

who desire only power or knowledge modify the masculine ideal. In fact, most people have a masculine goal or an equivalent of a masculine goal.

The masculine goal is, of course, only a fiction which determines what is " above " and what " below ", and enables the individual to select a guiding line. Every child creates many pairs of contrary concepts of " above " and " below ", as his own experiences in life suggest. Even normal children want to be tall and strong and take command in something—" like father,"—and this final goal influences their behaviour. Any child who feels small and helpless may accept the guiding fiction that he should behave as if his rôle was to be superior to everybody.

The neurotic is not alone in trying to make his life conform to fictions which increase his sense of personal importance. The healthy person also would have to give up all hope of orientation in the world if he did not try to make his picture of the world and his experiences conform to fictions. These fictions assume very definite shape in times of uncertainty, and find expression in the individual's opinions, beliefs and ideals.

The fiction of a final goal of power attracts all human beings, especially people who feel uncertain of themselves, such as neurotics. The influence of this fictive goal is enormous. It draws all psychic forces in its direction.

[63]

THE FICTIVE GOALS

A human being's fictive goals and the guiding lines by which he hopes to reach his goals remain unchanged throughout his life as long as they are not disclosed by unusually penetrating self knowledge. That he must have if he is to change them. A human being's character is the outcome of his life plan, fictive goals and guiding lines. Passions and " instincts " are exaggerated characteristics. An apparently spontaneous change of character may occasionally be observed, but if it was not due to the exercise of an unusual degree of insight, or to external influences, such as a change of environment, it generally proves to have been superficial. The most cherished goals were not abandoned. Consequently the fundamental nature of the personality remained unaffected. The change was merely a change in the choice of means.

[64]

CONSCIOUSNESS AND CONSCIENCE

THE ordinary man has very little idea of how his own mind works. He does not know that all his actions betray a bias although this is plain to an onlooker. We are thus brought face to face with a remarkable fact :—that it is possible for an individual to have " unconscious " tendencies, inclinations and motives.

The modern craze for psycho-analysis has so popularized the word " unconscious " that every one now uses it without realizing what complicated problems the concept involves.

Consciousness is a faculty of the mind that is comparatively easy to understand. Man has the capacity for " knowing " much of what goes on in his mind. Apparently this knowledge, which we call " consciousness ", is connected with functions performed by certain parts of the brain. But not only has it been pointed out that these parts of the brain represent nothing more than a disappearing portion of the whole, an observation which in itself does not take us far, as it seems probable that large sections of the human brain fulfil no functions ; it has also been ascertained that the functions fulfilled in the centres of consciousness constitute only an insignificant part of all the activities of the human

[65]

CONSCIOUSNESS AND CONSCIENCE

brain. That is to say, consciousness is only one of the many functions of the human brain. At the same time we have every reason to believe that our capacity for conscious thought develops with the development of speech. There is a close connection between language and conscious thought, for conscious thought is always symbolic thought. We can hardly conceive of consciousness without symbols or words.

What on the other hand is the unconscious ? Shall we be right in applying the term " unconscious " to everything that goes on in the human brain beyond the grasp of consciousness ? Hardly ; for as a rule our consciousness is able to hold only one or at the most a few thoughts, while our brain fulfils a great variety of functions. Countless impressions reaching our sense organs set in motion reflex processes and many activities follow automatically without any thought on our part.

We had to learn many every-day accomplishments before we became expert in them. There is no doubt that skill in these accomplishments, whether they involve physical movements or intellectual activities, was acquired only by the exercise of particularly keen powers of observation, which were, in fact, cortical in origin. As training in a brain process goes on, a centre is fixed for the whole co-ordinated complex, which gradually becomes embedded in the sub-cortical.

Walking, for instance, involves countless mus-

[66]

CONSCIOUSNESS AND CONSCIENCE

cular movements, which we no longer have to control, because they merge into each other and form a unit. So walking is an acquired accomplishment which we can use at will. When we are learning a language we try to master and understand single words, learn phrases and repeat sounds. We then have a certain vocabulary, we can express ourselves, we can pronounce words and we have gained powers which we exercise automatically when we wish to use the language. Is it reasonable to include all these brain processes, which are performed without our consciousness, in the term " unconscious " ?

Before attempting to answer this question we will examine the meaning given to this word " unconscious " by popular usage. People do not, of course, use the term " unconscious " to describe everything of which they know nothing, but they talk of having done certain definite things unconsciously. In fact, ever since the word was popularized—chiefly by Freud—people have talked about " the unconscious " when they might have expressed what they meant more simply by saying, " I ought to have known this, but actually I knew nothing about it." They therefore use the word " unconscious " to describe any psychological or mental process which, as experience shows, normally comes within the grasp of their consciousness, but in this special instance is hidden from their knowledge.

[67]

CONSCIOUSNESS AND CONSCIENCE

So the quality of " the unconscious " characterizes above all inclinations and tendencies which are not known to us. In everyday life we are aware of the part played by our consciousness chiefly in making plans and in carrying out our wishes. Conscious thought prepares the way for action.

Nevertheless, modern psychological research shows that even in preparing the way for action consciousness does not play such a decisive part as was formerly supposed. The behaviour of the smallest child is a study in discrimination. He knows what he wants, realizes what the consequences of certain kinds of behaviour will be and correctly gauges situations which are often very complicated—all this at an age which certainly excludes the possibility of his having any consciousness in our sense of the word, that is, power to think symbolically, for he may still be in his infancy.

Nor can we very well speak of " unconscious " processes where consciousness has not yet developed. We must have this contrast between " the conscious " and " the unconscious " before we can form an idea of either. It is unreasonable to suppose that " the unconscious " can exist where consciousness is lacking. Consciousness dawns only with the development of a thinking, knowing personality. And now we come to the point where we must ask how an apparent cleavage of consciousness originated.

[68]

CONSCIOUSNESS AND CONSCIENCE

We have seen how the child's personality is developed by the part he plays in the human community, how he may encounter difficulties when he tries to get himself accepted as a member of the community and how he may fail to respond in a positive way to his environment. Many of his actions are stratagems which he employs in a struggle against his environment. The child's guardians generally fail to understand most of these stratagems. They do not trace them back to their real causes, but think that they indicate faults for which the child is to be held blameworthy. The guardians' influence is generally limited to impressing on the child the fact that his behaviour is wrong without helping him to change his attitude. As long as the child rejects the guardians' principles he is free to rebel against them. His obstinate and defiant behaviour is entirely consistent. The grown-ups, however, have so much power that the child dare not resist them openly. He therefore has to behave as if he means to obey his guardians, especially if he wants their help. This is when conscience begins to develop. Conscience implies no more and no less than acceptance of the rules and principles represented by the guardians.

All children know perfectly well what is expected of them and what the established rules are. Most children accept these rules if only as a matter of form because it is too dangerous and difficult to defy them. For open defiance the child substitutes a

CONSCIOUSNESS AND CONSCIENCE

struggle within himself and in this the guardians generally encourage him because they hope that exercise of " self control " will lead to the final victory of " good " in the child. Naturally this type of upbringing is never successful. The child's hostile and negative impulses are unchanged, even though they may be concealed beneath an appearance of good intentions.

This situation, which arises in childhood, changes very little during the remainder of the individual's life. At first conscience represents only the guardians' wishes. Later it seems to personify law and order in the community. Conscience indicates awareness of the claims of the community, and in so far as the individual is the product of a " good " education his conscience accepts these claims. But whenever he obeys motives which reveal hostility to the community and a desire for personal superiority he becomes involved in a conflict with himself. Every part of his ego which represents the standpoint of general morals appears to range itself against actions instigated by asocial tendencies. At this moment when he appears to have renounced singleness of purpose and has to choose between two incompatible objectives he takes the same line of conduct which he adopted with success when he ranged himself as a child against his guardians. He makes excuses.

At first excuses were intended to pacify the guardians and ward off or mitigate punishment.

[70]

CONSCIOUSNESS AND CONSCIENCE

After the education of the conscience had proceeded further and the individual had himself become convinced of the justice of the rules he had been taught he found it necessary to excuse himself before his own conscience. His best way to do this is simply to repudiate responsibility for his own evil and unnatural inclinations—in fact, to know nothing about them. So the unconscious is created.

The unconscious embraces all emotions, wishes and inclinations for which people will not be responsible, or which they will not admit they have, in order to evade responsibility. It is not limited, as Freud thinks, to " suppression " of sexual emotions. In the early days of Psycho-Analysis the sexual life perhaps appeared to be hedged about with special prohibitions. Nowadays people are far less unwilling to acknowledge their sexual desires than to recognize their own responsibility and the extent to which they arrange their own lives. The " unconscious " is not by any means the uncanny power it has been represented to be by Psycho-Analysis. " After all, nothing in life is entirely known and nothing entirely unknown."[1] If people used instead of the word " unconscious " the more accurate word " unconfessed " they would simplify a problem which they otherwise make very confusing.

[1] Adler.

[71]

THE UNITY OF THE PERSONALITY

PRACTICALLY everyone divides the ego into two parts, ranging " I must " against " I ought not " and emphasizing the contrast between " I will " and " I cannot ". Invariably this contrast is created by self-deception. It is the excuse of a man who wants to absolve himself from responsibility, whether in the eyes of others or in his own eyes, for a certain action or a certain line of conduct. His purpose in having an inward conflict at all is to exculpate himself and make it seem that while he means well his own weakness, due either to constitutional defects or inherited faults of character, prevents him from carrying out his good intentions. In reality the united personality with its consistent purposiveness underlies and transcends all apparent contradictions.

The doctrine of the unity of the personality gave Individual Psychology its name. This name, which is so often misunderstood, is derived from the Latin word " individuum," which literally means " undivided," " indivisible " (in-dividere). " Individual variety " is the outcome of the life style, which varies with every single individual and is characteristic of him alone. His life style is based

[72]

UNITY OF PERSONALITY

on consistent purposiveness, which assigns a special place in the whole plan to every one of his actions. Contradictions in the same person, and that apparent duality which we think we observe in ourselves and others form part of a consistent mode of behaviour.

Inconsistencies and bipolarity invariably characterize the thoughts and actions of a person who has no intention of proceeding openly towards his goal. The possibility of reaching the same goal by following diametrically opposed lines of conduct accounts for the bewildering changes he makes in his behaviour in order to evade tasks and conceal his irresponsible tendencies.

Whether the child is defiant or obedient his object is the same—to assert the value and importance of his personality and to win an advantage over the grown-ups. His defiance gives the grown-ups a direct proof of their helplessness. His obedience makes use of them and compels them to help him.

A man who fears women because he does not feel able to cope with them will either become a hater of women and run away from them, or assume the character of a Don Juan in order to play off one woman against another.

Either too much or too little ardour may stand in the way of fulfilment of a task and make it possible to evade the task together with the danger of a defeat. Contradictions in the same person

[73]   F

UNITY OF PERSONALITY

involving a struggle between incompatible feelings and wishes serve a common purpose. These apparent contradictions may be necessary to achieve the intended result as in the following fable :[1]

A traveller going along a country road overtakes two tramps. One of them gets into conversation with the traveller and goodnaturedly gives him information about the roads which lie ahead, short cuts he could take and the best inns to stop at. Meanwhile the other tramp uses the opportunity to pilfer something from the traveller's bag. Later on when the traveller discovers the theft he will not fail to realize that the two tramps were accomplices, in spite of the apparent difference in their behaviour.

The person who clings to hesitation between two tendencies or inclinations is generally trying to reach a negative goal, not openly but by cunning, and the purpose of his contradictions is to hide his goal from his own conscience. Anyone who feels strongly attracted by two people and cannot decide between them is holding aloof from both, but nevertheless gives the impression of wanting to make up his mind. Often when people halt between two decisions they are merely trying to gain time and postpone making any decision at all.

The previous chapter discussed the significance of all inward conflicts. When only unimportant

[1] For which I am indebted to Dr. Horvat, Abbazia.

UNITY OF PERSONALITY

issues are involved, these conflicts provide opportunities for making romantic gestures, for often people who have deserted from the firing line of life fly to a minor seat of war, where they content themselves with false glory won in battles which are more spectacular than serious. A man who is skilful in arranging conflicts with his feelings may attach great importance to a very minor and matter-of-course detail of decent behaviour, because it makes him proud of his " self-control ". Actually he may have no reason for being extraordinarily proud of winning victories over his own feelings. For instance he shows no particular merit in not indulging in certain luxuries if he has other more urgent calls on his purse. But how much nobler he seems to himself if he has to struggle for a long time with his irrepressible longing for luxuries before he can overcome it !

So every contradiction in individual purposiveness proves to be deceptive.[1] In order to discover the object pursued by a certain individual on a certain occasion it is, of course, necessary to know his special circumstances and above all to have an insight into his personality. The same actions and the same conflicts may involve very different issues for different people. Ideas, wishes and emotions throw far less light on the personality than actions.

[1] Even the community feeling and the inferiority feeling are not hostile forces which produce duality. Rather they are to be regarded as two co-ordinating factors which characterize all behaviour.

UNITY OF PERSONALITY

Under certain circumstances we may indeed consider that thoughts and feelings have the value of actions. On the other hand thoughts, feelings and above all wishes very often contradict what is actually done. Actions are the only safe guide for understanding the personality, which so often turns towards fictive goals. We must make up our minds to regard everything else as mere embroidery. In fact, all wishes and feelings that contradict actions are misleading.

Power to appreciate the significance of actions not only helps us to build up a technique for studying human nature. It is most valuable in connection with self-education. Particularly in our own lives we find that apparent contradictions in our thoughts, emotions and wishes, occupy the foreground of our consciousness, so that we forget to judge our actions. The reason why self-knowledge is so difficult to acquire is that for the sake of maintaining an ethical personality we try to hide any of our impulses which are hostile to society from ourselves. Further, true self-knowledge would bring us disconcerting revelations. Our own fictive goals would be disclosed. We should see that they were mistaken goals and they would have to be given up. But an apparent splitting of the personality makes it possible for us to reconcile the real claims of environment with the imaginary claims of will-to-power.

[76]

NEUROSIS

THE lives of neurotics are full of contradictions between wishes and actions. Wherever we find neuroses we find that these contradictions appear to be based on the idea of illness. A human being's free control over himself and his actions and his powers of endurance appear to be as much restricted by a nervous illness as by a physical injury. Yet no direct physical correlation corresponds to the nervous symptoms. In fact, the organism is healthy. Any somatic changes which can be traced objectively are limited to the vegetative system. This, however, is nothing more than an apparatus for regulating physical functions, which can also be controlled by the mind. All the physical symptoms of neurosis are created by mental tension. Further, any pathological changes in the vegetative system can be explained in the same way.

We cannot disregard the fact that in the neurotic we have a healthy man who gives the impression of being ill and undeniably exhibits symptoms of illness, with the result that it is not always easy in making a diagnosis to distinguish between a " merely " nervous and a " real " illness.

Here we have yet another example of man's

[77]

NEUROSIS

capacity for deceiving himself and others by constructing false analogies. We have seen how he dissociates himself from his own will as soon as a contradiction between his wishes and actions appears to offer some advantage. Neurotic illness draws an analogy between itself and physical pain, which really does restrict physical functions quite independently of the will. So the neurotic (though, of course, without admitting it) uses his unimpaired will power to reproduce symptoms of illness which enable him to feel that his command over his will is restricted just as it would undoubtedly be by a physical illness.

The problem—how to arrange an illness " unconsciously ", that is to say, without admitting that it is arranged—was simplified chiefly by the teachings of Beard. These teachings, which were widely studied by experts and laymen, put forward the hypothesis of a nerve force said to be subject to disturbances. Beard sought to find some physical explanation for all symptoms nowadays described as nervous and called them illnesses of the nervous system or of " the nerves." But the existence of this hypothetical " nerve force " (which was said to be easily exhausted by overwork, excitement, sexual perversions and the strain felt by people who suffer from inherent weaknesses, with the result that nervous ailments or neurasthenia developed) could never be proved objectively. The limits of endurance could only be discovered subjectively

NEUROSIS

by each person for himself. So whenever an individual evaded tasks, his evasion was regarded as a form of illness which had developed because his nerve force was not sufficiently strong to bear the strain he put on it. These teachings so popularized the " contradiction " between what people can do and what they want to do, that anyone can now make use of the idea whenever it suits him. In fact, all that is needed once people have accepted this idea is that it should be possible for them to " learn " symptoms of illness. So a medical hypothesis, which otherwise would never have been taken seriously, rapidly won general acceptance in spite of its improbability.

There is always a definite moment when a nervous illness begins. This indicates that the individual is confronted with tasks which he does not feel able to perform, but the fact is not always very obvious, because the neurotic naturally tries to make out that the difficulties he encounters in life are the consequences and not the causes of his illness. Many neurotics even deny the existence of the difficulties they have, because they want to avoid the suspicion that their nervous symptoms serve a purpose. As most of us are ill prepared to perform the tasks of life, we easily become " nervy ".

Even a child has to bear special burdens and may develop "nervosity". This frequently finds expression in the so-called impossible behaviour of troublesome and difficult children. When a second

[79]

NEUROSIS

child is born or school life begins a very spoilt child is suddenly confronted with tasks for which he has had no training whatever. His courage may be taxed even more severely by a change in his environment or the death of his mother. If he then tries to escape from all test situations and evade many claims, the first nervous symptoms will probably appear. These may take the form of various disturbances of organ functions—difficulties affecting the digestive organs, like enuresis. Fits of panic and rages are also nervous symptoms. They are intended to serve a definite purpose, namely to compel the parents to give in to the child and to relieve him of certain tasks. They are the weapons which the child uses to get his own way.

Fear in particular is a weapon which is employed at some time or other by practically all children. Children find it easiest to enlist the parents' help by emphasizing their own weakness. A spoilt child who has not much confidence in his own powers is so easily alarmed that he gives way to wild panic the moment the slightest burden is laid on him—though it may amount to no more than being left alone for a short time. In any nervous illness he develops in adult life he will probably make some use of the weapon of fear which he learnt to use in childhood. This explains why fear plays such a large part in the lives of most neurotics.

[80]

NEUROSIS

Occasionally even school children have nervous breakdowns. Just before they are to take an examination they become overwrought ; they cannot sleep ; their minds grow confused ; they have trembling fits and develop all the symptoms of what is known as neurasthenia. Many people go on dreaming about school examinations long after they have grown up. Just as at school their abilities were tested by examinations they believe ever after that their abilities are always about to be tested by life or the human community. All that is tested in reality is our community feeling and our readiness to co-operate. Only the person who gives his co-operation subject to his cutting a good figure and who wishes to play no part which is not distinguished feels excessively alarmed about possibilities of failure and discredit.

A nervous illness always conceals a tendency to evade tests which life is bound to bring. The purpose is to safeguard the neurotic against the danger of discovering his own lack of value. At first this sounds like a paradox. For just because his nervous state makes him feel so weak and miserable his incapacity in many fields is rendered conspicuous. But remarkable as it may sound, he derives a fictive increase of value from his incapacity, for he consoles himself for his failures by saying : " If only I weren't such a bundle of nerves . . . if only I weren't so unfortunate as to be ill, then . . ." Whatever happens he must

[81]

NEUROSIS

preserve his idea of his own value. So though his capacities are unimpaired, he will not allow them to be tested. He makes his illness responsible for his undeniable failures, but his fiction about himself is the great obstacle to achievement. Further, while he excuses himself for achieving nothing he increases the demands he makes on those around him. Because he feels ill he not only considers that he is released from obligations to others (obligations involved in professional, social and love relationships), but also thinks that he is entitled to more consideration, more sympathy and more help from his friends and family.

The more discouraged a man becomes and the less fitted he feels to fulfil the requirements of life, the more determined he will be to evade the life tasks. His inclination to take refuge in a nervous illness is planted long before the actual appearance of symptoms of any kind. The moment the symptoms arise it becomes evident that community feeling has reached its limits and that a mistaken life plan has come into collision with the real conditions of life. No one can tell how much a pupil has learnt until his knowledge is tested. Those whom life subjects to difficult tests may come to the limits of their community feeling sooner than others who do not have to undergo the same tests. But in any life any lack of community feeling must sooner or later be revealed owing to the multiplicity and complexity of the relationships which human

[82]

NEUROSIS

co-operation in any task involves. Therefore difficulties encountered in life do not necessarily evoke nervous symptoms. Frequently very real difficulties change the condition of a neurotic not for the worse, but for the better. For as the purpose of nervous complaints is chiefly to provide excuses, they become superfluous as soon as external difficulties seem to condone evasion. Alarming nervous trouble often disappears at the beginning of a severe physical illness, that is to say, if the new illness serves as an excuse for retreat.

The neurotic is always an ambitious person who has lost courage. He lives in constant dread of his weaknesses being discovered and all his actions show that he is afraid. He has a typically hesitating attitude. As far as possible he avoids making up his mind about anything. So he postpones decisions, either to gain time, or to preserve his fictitious security at least for a moment. He tries to hold aloof from other people and from tasks for more than one person, because he doubts whether without special safeguards he can maintain himself at all. His life is one long struggle. The tension of his mind never relaxes. He is always on the alert in case he should be attacked. He sleeps uneasily and is often troubled by alarming dreams. His inner tension may also be betrayed by purely physical symptoms, by the blinking eyelids, trembling fingers, reflex hyperexcitability and exaggerated irritability and lability of the vaso-

NEUROSIS

motor nerves which characterize most neurotics. And because the neurotic is extremely excitable and sensitive, he responds readily to the most various suggestions. He is always keyed up. Just as a balloon filled with air rebounds violently at every touch, he makes the maximum response to every influence.

Tension plays a very important part in the development of symptoms. Without tension most of them would never appear at all. The symptoms assume forms as various as man's functions, any of which can be disturbed either by excesses or by neglect. The neurotic taking a subjective view of himself may even see disturbances where there are none, because he expects or wants to find less strain in the use of one function or more in the use of another, to break down a difficulty here or set up an obstacle there.

Having worked himself up to a state of tension he engages in a sham fight with himself, that is to say, with the functions of his body, his motor system, his feelings or thoughts. He has no difficulty in collecting symptoms. A person can lie awake a whole night without regarding this as an illness, but if he gets angry or very anxious about it or is thrown off his balance in any way, he begins to feel ill. His struggle with himself steadily increases the tension, without which he would never have begun it. The tension itself was first produced when he began to fight against his fellow

[84]

NEUROSIS

beings. It grows out of resentment and resistance to the requirements of life and above all out of fear of discredit and defeat. If the first symptoms produced by the struggle are suppressed they serve to increase the tension, which ultimately finds an outlet through an increasing number of new symptoms.

If nervous troubles affect a certain organ they always reveal themselves in disturbances of the function of the organ ; all organ neuroses are produced by tension. The increased strain makes itself felt first through the regulating apparatus of the vegetative nervous system and the internal secretory glands which are directly controlled by the mind.

Organ neuroses are often connected with an organ inferiority. This may be constitutional or may have been produced by faulty use of certain organs. We still know far too little about the importance of the child's attitude to his functions in life for regulating all organs through the vegetative system—even in the pathological sense. But we know that a functional inferiority of the digestive system may be produced either in response to a constitutional organ inferiority or by the use made of the organ in a struggle between a child and anxious parents, who attach special importance to plentiful meals and precautions intended to aid digestion.

This applies to all other nervous troubles. There

NEUROSIS

may be a disturbance of any function. Only a training varying in length is necessary to produce the disturbance. Organ inferiorities may make the process of training easier and influence the choice of symptoms. What, however, decides the choice of symptoms is not merely the ease with which they can be produced, but the adequacy of the symptom complex to provide excuses. For as every neurotic is trying to evade some task, this is, of course, the factor which decides what symptom is chosen. An accident may influence the neurotic's choice by calling his attention to the suitability of a symptom.

All views of neurosis which take the symptom as a starting point are superficial. The various forms of neurosis, hysteria, neurasthenia, anxiety neurosis, compulsion neurosis, mania, organ neurosis and sexual neurosis differ from each other only in the symptoms they select. The inward form of the neurosis is always essentially the same. Identical symptoms should never be attributed to identical causes, in view of the multiplicity of the factors which influence each person. It is of primary importance to discover what opportunities the individual had in childhood for producing neurotic symptoms, and how long the neurotic training has lasted. People can soon " cultivate " sleeplessness, forgetfulness, headaches, fits of depression, excitement and panic. A longer training is required for more serious nervous disturbances affecting the

[86]

NEUROSIS

circulation, the action of the pulse, palpitations of the heart and erytrophobia. The longest training of all—a training which generally begins in childhood and is continued without interruption—is required for developing compulsion neurosis.

Here at the very beginning the compulsion exerted by the human community and represented by the parents is counteracted by the compulsion under which the child places himself and which he apparently has to obey at an early age. This compulsion ranges itself against the human community. As a rule compulsion neurotics, who override all the claims of other people, regard themselves as unusually agreeable and interesting. For this reason it is very difficult to treat them. Naturally they stoutly resist any attempt to make them recognize that their behaviour is not the outcome of a painful illness, but of a cleverly concealed hostility to their fellow beings arising out of their special need for significance. For with this revelation the whole life plan of these people would fall to pieces.

The neurotic's tendency to hide his hostile impulses towards his fellow beings helps him to carry on a sham fight with his symptoms. Actually, as we saw, the tension thus produced aggravates the symptom complex. Another way of strengthening a neurotic line of conduct and of concealing the neurotic's own interest in the illness is provided by the feeling of pain. This becomes all the more

[87]

NEUROSIS

apparent the less the tendency to illness deceives others or the neurotic himself and the more he demands of other people on the plea of illness. Compulsion neurotics and hypochondriacs generally have the strongest subjective sufferings, since the community feeling, which causes people to acquiesce in social order, is most seriously injured by the style of life they adopt. Of course, if any other form of neurosis produces an equally violent disturbance, the suffering which ensues is equally severe. Pain and unhappiness always contain accusations against the world, and substitute for the sufferer's own responsibility the duty of others to help and comfort.

CRIME AND INSANITY

THE impulses which characterize both neurosis and crime grow out of hostility to the human community. But the hostility felt by the criminal appears to be very different from the hostility felt by the neurotic. Outwardly the neurotic remains a moral person, for he recognizes the rules of the human community, while the criminal is consciously and intentionally hostile to social order. It is not necessary for him to deceive himself regarding his tendencies for the sake of keeping a clear conscience. Nevertheless the criminal tries to shift the responsibility for his actions on to the community—on to other people. For even he is bent on safeguarding his idea of his value as far as possible. In fact, we find that many criminals are so proud of their exploits that they consider themselves better than people who appear to be more respectable. Above all, the criminal sets about an action in quite a different frame of mind from the neurotic's. He takes the line of active aggression. He goes straight for his goal.

If the criminal appears to be more courageous than the neurotic, his courage is of a strange order. It is not the courage which finds expression in useful achievements and makes contributions to the

CRIME AND INSANITY

community. It is the foolhardiness of a coward, who tries to conceal his secret despair by exhibitions of daring, and will not admit that he is afraid. It is the recklessness of an adventurer who stakes everything on one card. Superstition appeals to the imagination of gambler and criminal alike. Both believe against all probability that their plans will inevitably prosper. The only difference is that while the gambler claims the special favour of an impersonal destiny, known as luck, the criminal invokes this aid against the whole community, the laws and those who defend the community. The criminal also confines his exploits to a small arena. One proof that criminals lack courage is provided by the fact that they are all specialists. One specializes as a pickpocket, another as a burglar and another as a forger.

The criminal ranges himself against all the powers set up to defend law and order. He defies them just as he defied his guardians in childhood. If a child becomes so rebellious and resists his guardians so violently that he cannot be induced to accept the laws of order at least as principles of conduct, he will not place himself under any compulsion which will hamper him in fighting by developing a conscience. He has no qualms about using any weapons by which he may be able to wound his guardians. The very reason why he is so free from all restraints is that he does not need to excuse himself before his own conscience, whereas the

[90]

CRIME AND INSANITY

" nervous " child, who puts up a fight with himself, makes no more than an indirect attack on social laws and other people.

When the child makes no secret of his hostility to society he grows hardened. He resents correction, begins to tell lies and perhaps to steal, for in these ways he appears to triumph over his guardians. Yet people ought to realize that practically all children make a few small experiments in lying and stealing, which provide special opportunities for teaching them the rules of social order. Therefore wrong treatment by guardians, who dishearten the child about such faults and deny that he has any good intentions or feelings whatever, helps the child on the path to crime. On the other hand, even when an anti-social attitude has already been adopted, love and confidence can awaken the dormant spirit of co-operation in the child.

For even the criminal is not devoid of all community feeling. On the contrary he evinces community feeling in the way he behaves to his confederates. He often forms close social relationships within his own particular group and is even prepared to sacrifice himself for this group. But the group also has cut itself adrift from the great human community—in fact, only hostility to the community as a whole keeps it together.

Further, the criminal finds it impossible to avoid contact with the community. His character shows

[91]

CRIME AND INSANITY

the effect of the impression he has received that he has been forced to go in a certain direction because he was convinced that he had been personally repulsed by the community. He could only become a criminal after he had given up trying to win a position within the community and compensate for his feeling of weakness by means of useful achievements.

Inordinate ambition plays a decisive part in a criminal's life. His sole object in fighting is to gain significance. So people who break laws for other reasons, such as want, philosophical motives, etc., never develop the uncompromising character of the confirmed criminal. The true criminal wants to prove that he is cleverer than the community. He prides himself on being able to outwit the police. Every criminal acts on the assumption that he will not be caught. This alone makes a career of crime seem romantic and causes the confirmed criminal to run the greatest risks of punishment. Even the death penalty fails to deter him.

By resisting social order the criminal becomes an outlaw living outside the community and contenting himself with achievements on the useless side of life. Similarly the insane person cuts himself adrift from the community by denying the reason and logic of the community's laws. While the criminal substitutes the group formed by his confederates for the community he attacks, the psychotic creates a world which has nothing to do

CRIME AND INSANITY

with reality. He tries to gratify his desire for importance in this fantastic world because he has given up trying to assert himself in the real world. The psychotic therefore represents discouragement in its most terrible form. He gives up pretending to take the slightest interest in useful achievement. He severs the last bond uniting him with other people. His mind no longer has anything in common with theirs, because he ignores reason— either in all his actions or only in some. Yet his capacity for making contact with other people is never quite destroyed. As soon as his environment ceases to counter his fictive goals he can behave like a normal human being.

This, of course, applies chiefly to insanity which is not purely organic in origin, above all to schizophrenia and hypochondria. " Even when a purely organic psychosis, such as creeping paralysis, breaks out it is possible to trace its connection with the patient's personal attitude to life problems."[1] We have not yet been able to discover in what sense organ inferiorities influence psychotics, nor to what extent their symptoms represent weapons employed by them in their struggle to assert themselves So far only a beginning has been made in the psychological understanding of insanity. But at least the characteristic symptoms of hypochondria, such as self-reprobation, depression, etc., are known to be means for attaining a fictive increase in value

[1] Schilder.

[93]

CRIME AND INSANITY

and for compelling other people to condone the patient's behaviour instead of condemning it.

Latterly Individual Psychology has not been alone in showing that in reality the psychotic's attitude to the community (embodying readiness to strive for a position in the community and to take over useful functions, or the contrary) more or less decides whether the illness can be cured or will become more serious. For the successful experiments carried out in connection with vocational therapy, which was introduced by Simon (Gütersloh) and has been taken up by many others, all point in the same direction. It is to be hoped that by means of close co-operation between institutional psychiatrists and psycho-therapists it will be possible for psychology to arrive at a complete understanding of psychosis.

[94]

UPBRINGING

THE importance of the child's attitude to life for developing the personality and for determining the lot of each human being is shown most plainly of all in the lives of people who are failures, misfits or minus types ; that is to say in lives where the natural development of personality has been frustrated by maladjustment leading to neurosis, crime or insanity. If we recognize the importance of attitude in this sense we must also recognize the special importance of upbringing. This alone can systematically influence the child's choice of attitude and, in fact, fundamentally determine it.

The potential value of upbringing is considerably underestimated, not only by many lay persons, but also by a large number of professional teachers. They do indeed think it possible by educational methods to mitigate certain faults and defects in the child's so-called innate character, but they deny that education can make any fundamental difference. In support of their view they say that the child very early develops a definite individuality and that the child's individuality so resists the influences of education that all the known methods of reward and punishment are useless.

Scepticism about the value of education generally

[95]

UPBRINGING

grows out of an error regarding the age at which the child begins to respond to educational methods. Enough has already been said to suggest that it is possible to begin educating the child, not as is thought only at the age when he becomes " reasonable ", but actually on the first day of his life. Getting accustomed to regular feeding hours, and learning to bear the unpleasantness of feeling hungry or wet represent educational tasks in the positive sense. Mistakes in training may be made even at this period by people who interfere with regular habits, spend too much time looking after the child, do not allow him to sleep long enough and rock him or carry him about whenever he cries. It is true that all children are not alike at birth and that the development of some may be affected by organ inferiorities and illnesses. But the final effect these troubles have depends chiefly on the treatment which the child learns to expect from those who bring him up.

Some of us may wonder why this pessimism regarding the possibilities of upbringing so often prevails even in circles interested in education. The explanation is found in the methods by which people generally try to train and educate children. Parents especially often show a very uncritical spirit in accepting these methods.

A number of so-called bad habits are found among children. We all know children who bite their nails, children who pick their noses, children who

[96]

UPBRINGING

hold themselves badly, children who have a magnetic attraction for dirt. An anxious mother will be heard scolding her child for one of these failings on an average of a hundred times a day. Although no success is achieved in this way, for on the contrary the child continues to practise the habit, it still does not occur to the mother that possibly her method is at fault. But we know that if she were to ask how she could most quickly accustom the child to an unpleasant habit like nose-picking she need only call out when the child chances to touch his nose, " Take your hand away— you mustn't do that ! "—and the child will take the very next opportunity to push his finger up his nose. Then if she only scolds the child often enough for subsequent repetitions of this action they will crystallize into a habit. We see therefore that the mother's scolding method is calculated to train the child in a bad habit.

Countless bad habits are formed by children as the direct results of the parents' stupidity. The commonest reason why a small child learns to masturbate is that the scolding method has been employed by the parents, who " try to teach the child better " if he once or twice chances to touch his genitals in a harmless way. If a child is not coaxed to eat there will be no difficulty about feeding him. Anyone who fails to realize how closely faults are connected with faulty methods will easily make the mistake of under-estimating

[97]

UPBRINGING

or even denying the potential value of upbringing. All that is actually proved by the failure of the scolding method is that the method itself is useless and even harmful, for instead of disarming resistance in the child, it creates and strengthens it.

More or less the same may be said with regard to most of the time-honoured methods of upbringing which are still widely employed. The commonest educational expedients are threatening and blaming, which, if they produce the desired effect at all, only produce it outwardly. Blame always tends to make the child less willing to improve, and threats only succeed in making him more headstrong.

The injurious effect of blame generally cuts very deep. If a child does anything wrong, that is to say, does anything which violates social order, or transgresses the rules of the community, it is because he has ranged himself against the community or because he no longer has any confidence in his own capacity for useful achievement. Otherwise he would not have acted wrongly. People misuse only those opportunities and capacities in regard to which they do not expect much from themselves. When the child is not hampered by an inferiority complex he accomplishes useful things, or learns to accomplish them gradually. But blame only convinces the child that he was right to doubt his capacity in a certain direction. It does not strengthen—rather it weakens his belief

[98]

UPBRINGING

in his own powers, on which his success depends. The net result of scolding may easily be that a fault, far from being eradicated, takes firmer root. When a child is always being called dirty or stupid he will feel more and more convinced of his inferiority and find it increasingly difficult to act under any other assumption. Yet practically everyone who has to bring up children seems to think that some good result can be achieved by scolding and humbling them. These methods are also applied by grown-ups to each other. They believe that this treatment will influence people in the way they wish, and make them conform to some apparently desirable educational standard. It remains for us to discover how they ever came to this conclusion.

All those who resort to scolding try to justify their method on the ground that it is necessary to show people their faults so that they can correct them. It is surprising that they have hitherto failed to realize that their purpose can hardly ever be achieved by the method they use, especially as there are other more effective ways of pointing out faults. For instance, they could make a child aware of a fault by pointing out the difference between good and bad. Not, however, as is usually done, by pointing out how well behaved and clever some other child is. No good is done by telling Jack to " see how nicely Tommy works ! " A better plan is to emphasize the good in Jack

[99]

UPBRINGING

himself by saying to him " I am glad you have been working so well to-day." Even if there is a danger that Jack's devotion to work during the day has not after all been conspicuous, he himself knows that he has not tried as hard as he might have done. If a child has execrable handwriting, instead of remarking how badly he has written an exercise—which he probably sees for himself—it would be better to notice how well he has written one page, one line, one word or even only one letter. In this way the difference between what is ugly and what is beautiful, what is good and what is bad, is made quite plain to the child without discouraging him, because he is made to feel that he really could write better.

Therefore the reason for the popularity of scolding cannot be that it shows people their faults so that they can correct them. Rather, scolding betrays an unconscious tendency to disparage others. The fact is that parents and teachers frequently under-rate children and regard them as weak, helpless, stupid, clumsy, mischievous and perverse. Few parents know that their children—in early child-hood at least—are often better or more valuable human beings than they are themselves, simply because the children have not yet become so discouraged as the adults. Often the children are cleverer than their teachers. They pursue their objectives with much more decision and above all much more successfully. They search in every

UPBRINGING

direction for ways of reaching their goals, while the grown-ups generally confine their choice to a very limited number of ways and therefore cannot expect much success. Perhaps this is why adults are so ready to scold and disparage children.

Very often, also, the parents and teachers do not feel able to cope with their charges. They feel their responsibility towards the children but have no faith in their influence over them, and realizing how little they are fitted for their task of bringing up children, they behave like most people in difficult situations. They put the blame for their own failure and evasion on others. They undervalue the children in order to be able to keep up the fiction of their own superiority which is threatened by their failures. The naughtier a child is, the more the blame for the negative result of upbringing appears to lie with the child himself. So whenever the adults feel unable to deal with a child they content themselves with fixing the blame on the child and employ numerous " educational " methods against the child, threatening, correcting, scolding, forbidding and punishing without any good effect.

The bad educator is characterized by his fussiness and passion for meddling. He wants to show what a lot of trouble he takes, so that in the event of the child turning out a failure no share of the blame will fall to him.

People living in communities, husbands and

UPBRINGING

wives, members of the same households, people sharing authority, people in subordinate positions, workmates and club members, all treat their fellow human beings in the same way as soon as they feel weaker than them and unable to cope with them. Anyone who feels able to win recognition from others and does not believe that his prestige is endangered by others never grasps at such weapons.

Fault finding and scolding are only palmed off as educational methods. In reality they do not serve any educational purpose. Educators employ them merely in order to save their personal prestige.

But there are other quite different educational methods which really can help the children to develop their capacities. These methods are not content with exacting a show of obedience by the exercise of main force ; they can train self-reliant, capable and happy people. The whole purpose of education is to fit the child to take part in life with others and to help him to win and hold a position in the community—in other words, the purpose of upbringing is to develop the community feeling on which success and happiness in life depend.

This purpose is fulfilled automatically if the family as a whole is united and each member willingly and as a matter of course subordinates himself to the whole. The result of this kind of training is that from the very outset the child responds readily to the community, has a place of

[102]

UPBRINGING

his own and fulfils a function, which certainly differs from the functions of the grown-ups, but does not for this reason seem to be less valuable or important. We can be sure that we shall never find problems of upbringing and nervous people in a united family.

Unfortunately in these days ideal families are rare, especially in large towns. As a result education now has to contend with greater difficulties ; it is always having to remedy mistakes already made. If a child shows signs of being neurotic or is said to be a " problem " child, the greatest care has to be exercised in order to avoid mistakes which emphasize the difference between the child and other members of the community. Whenever a child begins to retreat in any direction this is a sign that he is beginning to lose faith in himself, and that he feels that he has been repulsed in some way by the community—owing to an organ inferiority, spoiling, snubbing or discouraging experiences he has had in his relationships with friends, a brother or a sister or other people. We ought to make it our first care to encourage a child when he is in difficulty. All the child's mistakes are manœuvres which he makes in his struggle against his environment and we cannot expect to check his fighting spirit if we ourselves join battle. Rather, we must come to terms with him.

It would be a great mistake, however, to suppose that the only way of keeping on good terms with

[103]

UPBRINGING

the child is by constantly giving in to him. This will not help the child who has taken up a position outside and against the family to find his proper place in the community. Praise and encouragement on the other hand can help him. (Of course, we must not according to a far too common parental practice tickle the child's ambition and urge him to achieve conspicuous successes. A child who is always being pushed is reduced at last to utter despair.) Once the social order has been disturbed the child will never find his place in the community unless those responsible for his training observe the following principle : he must bear the consequences of his own asocial behaviour. We ought to begin to apply this principle long before the child can talk—that is to say, while he is still in his infancy.

People who have to bring up children generally work on the opposite lines. They scold, humiliate and threaten—and the child gets his way after all. His weapons are generally more telling than theirs. He yells, becomes stubborn and defiant or cries. In the end they generally give in. They have too little patience to fight the battle out. So they would have done better to have avoided any clash of wills at all. If they only knew it they would not have to talk very much or threaten the child at all so long as they never tried to save him from the consequences of his own actions.

Some parents find it very difficult to deal with a

[104]

UPBRINGING

careless and untidy child. They threaten ; they try to make the child tidy by punishing and humiliating him—all in vain. In the end the mother herself has to put away the child's toys and the child is just as untidy as ever. How much simpler it is not to say anything at all and let the child learn for himself how tiresome it is not to be able to find things that he has not put away in their proper places.

Of course, when parents decide to let the child bear the consequences of his behaviour they must be a little bit cunning about it and sometimes look the other way and give him plenty of scope. Parents can learn all they need to know about cunning from their own children. There is no exhausting children's ideas for ways of outwitting parents and teachers, or the schemes they evolve for getting what they want.

Unreflecting people are not qualified to bring up children. Nobody should decide upon any educational method whatever—including any form of reproof or scolding—before considering all the possible effects and the feasability of other methods. It is vain to object that there is not sufficient time in everyday life for so much reflection. Reflection does not require as much time and energy as is now expended uselessly in education by people who go the wrong way to work. But the educator can train this capacity for reflection only by learning to do what is far from easy—to look on quietly

[105]

UPBRINGING

while the child makes experiments. Nowadays most educators suffer from anxious fear of neglecting something. They cannot bear to pass over any fault in silence. They feel that they must do something, and forthwith proceed to do something, even if it is worse than useless. If they would allow a child who has begun to retreat in a certain direction to take his way unchecked for a while, they would give him a chance to release pent-up feelings and their tolerance would considerably weaken his resistance, without which he could not persist in his faults.

This capacity for observing a fault quietly gives quite a different value to the educational methods that are finally selected. They are sure to have been well considered and will never involve the parents in a struggle for personal prestige. Often enough a simple explanation or a friendly discussion is sufficient to make a child realize the error of his behaviour. Of course, such a discussion should never be attempted, as unfortunately most often happens, immediately after the child has committed a fault, but only at a time when the child is feeling on friendly terms with his mentor—in quiet moments such as may occur during a walk.

These methods of upbringing do not make the child feel that he is being treated as a mere cipher. Consequently he is not impelled to resist the educators, but looks upon them as friendly guides, who accompany him while he takes his first steps

[106]

UPBRINGING

in life. Everything which stresses the authoritative position of the educators, will at the very least aggravate the child's want of self-reliance. More often, however, it creates bitter opposition. All forms of punishment, especially corporal punishment, and even rewards are very doubtful educational expedients, and should be replaced by the logic of an all-embracing order, which is not dependent on the arbitrary will of any single individual.

Good educators will respect the child's personality, love him well enough to understand his mistakes and show kindly firmness in refusing to save him from the unpleasant consequences of his own conduct. They will always find ways of reconciling the child to the social order without arousing his resistance. When the child becomes aware of the existence of the social order, they will help him to fit into it ; but they will not make the child feel that they wish to seize the opportunity to assert any claim to personal superiority or power. In addition, by judiciously encouraging the child they can help many capacities to unfold—capacities which most people still think can be developed only in unusually talented children. Training is all-important for developing any capacity or talent and we cannot yet even picture what kind of men and women will be produced in future times when different educational methods are employed.

[107]

UPBRINGING

In the days of large families the behaviour of the parents seems to have mattered less. A certain system of give and take automatically comes into being whenever a large number of brothers and sisters have to adapt themselves to each other. In a large family no child could help noticing mistakes in his own behaviour, and in this way much though not all of the damage caused by unsuitable educational methods was put right. At least the effects of many mistakes, from which all the children suffered equally, were mitigated.

In the small families of the present day the parents' mistakes have far more serious consequences, especially as people now feel much less certain as to how things should be done. They approach the very difficult task of education in a spirit of great uncertainty—all the more so because they now admit that bringing up children is an art which must be learnt like any handicraft, trade or profession. Unfortunately very few parents succeed in learning this art. They generally adopt the methods which they saw their own parents use, although they themselves suffered from them as children. As educational mistakes have been handed down from generation to generation their injurious effects have accumulated, with the result that at the present day education instead of helping the child to develop very often seriously discourages him. " A loveless upbringing may brand the child with the stigma of worthlessness. The

UPBRINGING

Draconic severity of a very harsh and strict upbringing intensifies the child's feeling of helplessness and dependency on the adults. A moralistic upbringing gives an appearance of serious depravity to the child's most insignificant mistakes. An upbringing characterized by constantly changing methods gives the child a feeling of utter insecurity. Educators who refuse to take the child seriously deprive him of his sense of responsibility. Discouragement always has an injurious effect on him. Coddling shelters him from experiences which develop his capacities."[1]

All that has been said in this chapter has referred mainly to upbringing in the every-day home milieu. More or less the same observations apply to community education in institutions, kindergartens and schools. Teachers can maintain order and impart knowledge without resorting to punishments and other repressive methods if they can help the child to fit into an organized and united community. Such a community will be sufficiently magnetic to draw even a child who at first resists it ; he can be persuaded to contribute without being compelled. The community feeling of the children, their instinct for the rules of social life, develop best in just these communities. Therefore children who are in danger of becoming ego-centric (like the only child, the youngest child, the spoilt child and the child whose upbringing has

[1] Ferdinand Birnbaum.

UPBRINGING

hitherto been loveless) should be brought into such communities as early as possible.

Individual Psychology has made the general technique of education easy to master. But school education freed from compulsive authority (which is an ideal after the hearts of Comenius and Pestalozzi) sets special new problems for teachers to solve patiently and gradually.

It may seem remarkable that the decisive factors which have to be considered in connection with education should never have been discovered by science until our day, for the art of bringing up children has been practised ever since there were human beings. Is it credible that wrong methods should always have been employed hitherto and that it should have been reserved for us to discover the right methods ? Here it may be helpful to call attention to an analogy in the history of medicine.

For many centuries all injured and wounded people who were taken into hospitals had their wounds bandaged with lint made from old linen rags. No one knew that this lint infected the wounds and produced complications which were fatal to large numbers of patients until Semmelweiss discovered the law of asepsis, and was able to prevent wounds from becoming infected. Before then people were actually nursed to their deaths by their well meaning helpers. We find a similar situation with regard to upbringing.

[110]

UPBRINGING

Educators whose duty it is to take care of the children injure them most dangerously without knowing or intending it by their wrong methods. It may be that the new teachings of Individual Psychology are destined to play just as revolutionary a part in education as the discoveries of Semmelweiss did in surgery and gynæcology. Then and not until then pessimism about upbringing, which may perhaps be justified under the present system, will be silenced.

PSYCHOTHERAPY

PEOPLE who have been brought up in the wrong way are very little fitted to fulfil the life tasks. They betray their wrong attitude to the human community by all the mistakes they make in their lives, by crime as well as by psychosis, and above all by neurosis. The only way to cure them is to help them to change their objectives and correct their attitude to their fellow beings. That is to say, therapy has to repair the damage done in childhood by faulty upbringing. Individual Psychology has given us a therapy which has been proved efficacious for treating both psychotics and criminals, but naturally the treatment of neurosis gives it the most scope.

All modern psychology is indebted to neurosis because it impelled philosophers and thinkers to make investigations which led to the discovery of the laws of psychic life. (It need not be objected that these laws apply to sick people only, because they were discovered by observing these people. In all branches of medicine we had to study the pathological organ before we could find out anything about the function of the healthy organ). Nervous people come the soonest to a psycho-

[112]

PSYCHOTHERAPY

therapist for treatment because from their standpoint there is something positively pathognomonic about the feeling of being ill. Success in psychological treatment depends on the therapist's power to make fearless co-operators in life out of timid and discouraged people. This suggests both the possibilities of psychotherapy and the difficulties with which the therapist has to contend.

If psycho-therapy is to be of any use at all it must give lasting encouragement. It can do this only by helping the patient to acquire self knowledge. Nobody need be a slave to his mistakes and wrong objectives if he can recognize his own responsibilities for them. The trouble is human beings find it extraordinarily difficult not to shirk their responsibility. Few people know themselves, though many pretend they do. Either they are too lazy to acquire self-knowledge or they habitually deceive themselves in order to hide their hostile tendencies towards their fellow beings and towards the whole community from their own consciences. Therefore true self knowledge is very rare. On the other hand it is just because people feel anxious to acquire it that modern psychological works awaken such widespread interest. By reading psychological books a man may become able to understand his fellow beings better and he may even learn to see through many of his own stratagems, but it is very difficult for him to acquire true self knowledge by reading only. Usually he needs

[113]

PSYCHOTHERAPY

to enlist the co-operation of somebody disinterested if he wants to understand his life plan, examine his fictive goals, extend his limited field of vision and see the true meaning of his actions and difficulties.

The earliest memories of his childhood and his dreams can take him a long way on his voyage of discovery. They show the direction in which he tends to go. The earliest memories of childhood are always significant. They record experiences in response to which the child developed his characteristic attitude and there can be no doubt that each individual tries to justify his attitude by looking back to those experiences. It often happens that if treatment succeeds in changing the patient's outlook, experiences he had kept in mind till then are forgotten and others which he had not been able to bring to mind take their place. All memories serve to justify a definite line of conduct which is being pursued at the time or has been planned for the future. The human being is constantly drawing on his memories for fresh strength to persist in a course once chosen.

His dreams serve the same purpose. They are like rehearsals showing how he intends to deal with the tasks of the immediate future. They strengthen his preference for retreat or pretence, and they help him to choose his tempo and direction. His dreams reveal many things which he will not confess while he is awake. This is why many people pay no

[114]

PSYCHOTHERAPY

regard to their dreams. If they understood their dreams they might find it difficult to keep up an appearance of self-confidence.

The doctor encourages the patient to tell what he remembers about his childhood and his dreams and invites his explanations of the situations of his childhood in order to understand the patient's everyday conduct and find out what type of person he is. Even the patient's attitude to the doctor provides an opportunity for observing how he behaves to his fellow beings.

The patient finds that chance has played a less important part in his life than he has imagined, as most of his experiences have been shaped by a plan. The patient is shown what plan he made when he prepared to approach life, and how much his experiences have turned on this plan. We shall find it easier to understand the important connection between the plan and actual experiences if we have noticed that when most cyclists first attempt to ride alone they often run into a stone or rut, although it really requires more skill to hit a small point in a wide space than to miss it. They have mistakenly made up their minds that they cannot avoid it and they act on this assumption.

Many people doubt themselves and give way to the feeling of not being able to act differently. This mistake is the origin of all faulty conduct and particularly all neurotic conduct. We can understand how as a child an individual arrived at a

[115]

PSYCHOTHERAPY

wrong answer when he tried to work out the problem of his own value and why he thought he was worth less than others in certain respects. It is the task of treatment to correct his mistake. Only new faith in his powers can induce the patient to give up safeguarding himself.

In essence any psychological treatment is an attempt to increase the patient's self confidence and to encourage him directly or—if the treatment is not on the lines of Individual Psychology—indirectly. Even exposure of the fraud which underlies the contradiction between what the patient " wants " to do and what he " can " do, between his apparent intentions and incapacity to give them effect, ultimately helps to encourage him. He sees that his failures have not been due to any deceptive weakness of character or equipment, but that he has been mistaken as to the nature of his intentions. The patient must recognize that the symptons upon which the illness has been built up are lines of retreat which he has prepared. Neurosis is like a mock battle field outside the war zone—a long way behind the front of life.

It is not sufficient for the patient to know how his personality has developed. The doctor must induce him to face the problems of his situation at the time of treatment (his " present problems ") while leaving him to make decisions for himself. Therefore the doctor's first objective is not to cure

[116]

PSYCHOTHERAPY

symptoms, but to persuade the discouraged patient to fulfil his tasks. The patient's difficulties never lie in the tasks themselves but arise out of his anxiety about his prestige and his dread lest a failure should prove his want of value.

In treatment the doctor has to try to overcome the patient's unwillingness to face unpleasant facts. A difficulty which always makes the problems of treatment more complicated is that the patient usually erects defences even against the doctor as he erected them against other people in childhood and has done ever since. The task of fundamentally changing the patient's life plan, which can only be performed by the doctor and patient together, is extraordinarily difficult and not at all pleasant for the patient. As nervous people tend to give up co-operating as soon as they have to do anything difficult, every patient tries a number of artifices in order to evade this task.

The patient does not always adopt an attitude of open resistance to the doctor. He can make himself just as inaccessible to treatment by indirect evasion. For instance, the patient's resistance may be expressed by an apparent tendency to fall in love with the doctor. The doctor then represents only a personal value. A rôle is allotted to him apart from his profession. The patient is interested in matters which have little to do with the treatment. Another form of evasion is practised by the patient who tries to ascribe the

[117]

PSYCHOTHERAPY

doctor's success to his personal influence. All forms of evasion, including the tendency to ascribe success or failure to the doctor alone, show that the patient is determined not to modify his own attitude to life nor to let himself be persuaded to set about fulfilling his own tasks by means of his own powers.

Here of course we can do no more than suggest the problems which complicate the task of the psycho-therapist. At least psycho-therapy gives the person whose community feeling has been insufficiently educated " another chance ". The doctor therefore has to play the rôle of educator. And like the educator he must avoid creating an impression of superior authority. He must never seem to be more than a sympathetic friend helping a discouraged person to recover his own self confidence. Otherwise he burdens himself with all the responsibility for the success or failure of the treatment, while in reality everything depends on how the patient responds. Determination to become community-minded and willingness to co-operate with others must put an end to the struggle for prestige in which the patient formerly engaged, because he contented himself with trying to overcome his feeling of inferiority in appearance only. There is no other cure for neurosis.

Neurosis is not a static indication of the extent to which an individual has failed to develop his community feeling. Rather it is dynamic, for it

[118]

PSYCHOTHERAPY

shows the direction in which he is moving, that is to say, that he is in retreat. The neurotic can be cured if only he can be induced to abandon his retreat from people and achievements. He cannot, of course, expect to be perfect. He can only change from greater to lesser error. Therefore a temporary relapse into neurosis need not be taken very seriously, unless the patient makes it a pretext for giving up the new direction he has adopted.

THE THREE LIFE TASKS

I

WORK

THE three life tasks, Work, Love and Friendship, may be regarded as representing all the claims of the human community. Ultimately right fulfilment depends on the development of community feeling and readiness to co-operate. Consequently if one of the tasks is evaded difficulties will sooner or later be experienced in fulfilling the others also. Occasionally it may seem as if one of the tasks is completely fulfilled, while no real effort is made to fulfil the others. The most striking examples of this apparent inconsistency are found in the different ways in which the same individual seems to regard the tasks of work and love, but closer examination reveals conflict and uncertainty and a very superficial and insecure feeling of happiness beneath all the apparent harmony. In the end the apparent success and evasion can always be reduced to a common denominator. The consistent life plan invariably decides whether and how any achievement is to be attempted or evaded.

Any apparent inconsistency in fulfilling the

[120]

WORK

three life tasks results partly from differences in the demands they make on the community feeling which is necessary for their fulfilment. Most people half fulfil the occupational task. Only the most discouraged people evade it, which is why inability to work is often regarded as being in itself a symptom of a serious illness. Of the three tasks the occupational task is still the most important for the maintenance of life, and nonfulfilment of it almost imperils existence. Some people devote practically the whole of what capacity for co-operation they have to fulfilling the occupational task. Also, though they could not do their work if other people did not co-operate with them, they are able to maintain a certain distance in their relationships with their fellow workers, for few people express their whole personality in their work. The more demand the work makes on the whole personality the more plainly every defect of personality is betrayed.

Occupational work may be defined as any kind of work which is useful to the community. It is by no means restricted to work which is remunerated by a wage or its monetary equivalent, but includes the work of the housewife and voluntary worker at welfare centres, provided that such work is not done at irregular intervals as the individual alone sees fit, but according to a certain system. The ultimate test is whether or not useful work is done for the community. Under our present social

[121]

THE THREE LIFE TASKS

system recognition of work most often takes the form of monetary remuneration. On the other hand the money paid to a shareholder corresponds to no kind of occupational work. But we shall be justified if we include preparation for a trade or profession in our definition of occupational work.

As occupational work is characterized by the value it has for other people, it seems to be connected with the idea of duty. It certainly deprives the worker of some opportunities to indulge his whims and inclinations which he had when he was not a worker. Apart from quite small children and old and infirm people there are few human beings whom special circumstances exempt from all occupational duties. All other people have some kind of work to do in the interest of their fellow beings, or have a certain necessary function to perform for the human community.

There are differences in the age at which different people begin to have work to do. Girls are usually given some duties to carry out for the family much earlier than their brothers. The more the child evades useful work the more difficult the occupational task appears. This applies to spoilt children whose duties the parents try to shoulder. On the other hand it applies with equal or even greater force to wilful and stubborn children who succeed in evading the duties allotted to them by their parents. By the national system of education, however, every child is compelled to face

WORK

the occupational task as soon as he becomes of school age.

The fact that we all have to take over duties does not mean that duty is necessarily characterized by everything that is disagreeable, as many people think. Duties should not supersede the child's games, but grow out of them in fulfilment of the laws of organic development. After all, games constitute a necessary preparation for practical life and in this way they are also connected with preparation for an occupation. Unless the whole upbringing is at fault it is easy to get the child to undertake duties which are harnessed to games. The apparent contradiction between games and duties exists only for adults, for the child takes his games at least as seriously as the adult his duties. It seems as if this contradiction must have been suggested by mistakes in upbringing. The child sensed that strong pressure was being brought to bear on him and resisted it, and finally allowed himself to be betrayed into a hostile attitude.

If hostility to duty develops during childhood, it generally persists in some form throughout the remainder of life. But it is not in the least necessary to feel resentful about duty. There are many people who derive a feeling of inward satisfaction and happiness from the fulfilment of duty in any form, including even the fulfilment of occupational tasks under difficulties, whilst other people cannot be induced to undertake any occupational tasks

[123]

THE THREE LIFE TASKS

no matter how pleasant the conditions of work may be. Ultimately readiness to take over occupational tasks depends on the individual's attitude to the community. He must be community minded if he is to find happiness in doing useful work in the community.

Difficulties in fulfilling the occupational task arise out of difficulties connected with the problem of personal prestige. We have seen how strongly a feeling of inferiority can affect the individual's attitude to the community. The more he is oppressed by a feeling of being weaker than the others, the more he will try in all he does to overcome it. He will do his utmost to influence events in a way which he thinks will help him to win greater significance. He will tend to think of his work less as a useful contribution to the community than as a circumstance which helps or hinders him in his struggle for prestige. The feeling of inferiority may be aggravated in occupations which are regarded as menial and in subordinate positions depending on the arbitrary authority and " prestige-hunger " of a capricious superior.

Many people are ready to put their hearts into their work only on one condition—that is to say, only when they feel that it involves no loss of prestige and their ambition is satisfied. They dislike their work as soon as they feel that their personal prestige is threatened, whether by

WORK

humiliations and slights of the most various kinds, or by possible failures which will prove that they are unfitted to do the work. No one who feels that he is being undervalued or exploited can feel happy in his work.

If a worker begins to evade the occupational task he does so either by skilfully and more or less "unconsciously" accumulating difficulties which make it impossible for him to go on working, or he will suddenly become quarrelsome and irritable and develop nervous symptoms which interfere with his work. These nervous symptoms are generally connected with mental functions—the capacity to concentrate and quickness of observation. They may be produced by sleeplessness or take the form of functional disturbances of the motor system, like the cramp which interferes with certain occupations, for instance, writer's cramp.

As a rule these methods of evading the occupational task are employed when failures threaten or have already occurred. Occasionally, however, we find an individual resorting to the same methods immediately after he has achieved an outstanding success if he thinks that people will now expect him to go on achieving successes on the same level and does not feel able to do so.

Even the crucial moments at which various types of people evade the occupational task are characteristic. Some break down just before they reach

[125]

THE THREE LIFE TASKS

their goal, others just after reaching it. This behaviour, which is typical of the individual and constantly recurs, can always be traced back to the idea that his personal prestige is at stake. Many people content themselves with insinuating that they could achieve special successes in some occupation but never attempt to achieve them because they are afraid that if they do their want of capacity will be revealed. It depends on how much courage they have whether they turn away from the path to achievement at the very beginning and make it plain that they have done so by constantly chopping and changing from one kind of occupational training to another, i.e., by hesitating between several occupations, or whether they face about just before they reach the goal of achievement. The worker who breaks down when he reaches the goal or after he has reached it is afraid of not being able to hold the position he has gained.

If any nervous or characterological disturbance interferes with an individual's work, he will not feel completely fit to work again until his life plan has been explained to him and his overweening ambition corrected by therapeutical treatment. Naturally, any ambition which he can satisfy without trespassing beyond the boundaries of useful achievement will not cause any disturbance in his life, but on the contrary will provide a special impulse for doing extremely valuable work.

[126]

WORK

While nonfulfilment of any of the life tasks is at once the expression of undeveloped community feeling and an experience which aggravates the feeling of inferiority, failure to fulfil the occupational task—that is to say, occupational unemployment is the heaviest burden any human being can have to bear. The burden of unemployment weighs most heavily on people who have met with failures in their love life and in their friendships. These people have no other effective way of keeping in touch with the community. They do not know how to feel useful except in their work. Some of them may have utilized excessive professional ambition as an excuse for evading the love task or for failing to form friendships. It is very understandable that they should feel that the involuntary termination of occupational employment owing to illness, reduction of staff or superannuation spells complete expulsion from the human community. Sundays and holidays have a similar deadening effect on some people. For when work no longer provides them with an outlet, their failures in love and friendship become all the more conspicuous.

[127]

II

LOVE

In contrast to the occupational task the love task is fulfilled comparatively rarely at the present time. On the one hand defective community feeling can more readily reveal itself in evasion of this task, because the consequences of evasion do not seriously limit the chances of maintaining life. On the other hand right fulfilment of the love task demands a maximum of community feeling, because it involves the closest of all contacts between two human beings, tests their capacity for co-operation to the utmost and destroys the distance which can always be preserved in occupational and social relationships. Further, fulfilment of the love task is bound up with special difficulties at the present time.

By right fulfilment of the love task is meant close union of mind and body and the utmost possible co-operation with a partner of the other sex. Such a solution of the problem can be reached only if each partner fully accepts the other and a feeling of mutual obligation grows up between them.

There are several reasons why this task appears to offer more difficulties nowadays than in the past

[128]

LOVE

and is fulfilled by only a small number of people. It is obvious that people are less courageous to-day than they were in the past. Their want of courage is due not merely to economic and social insecurity but also to the smallness of most present day families, for when there are only a few children the danger of spoiling is much greater. We have seen that the more discouraged people are the more value they set on what they regard as their prestige and the more desperately they fight for it. To-day the struggle between the sexes for prestige is more bitter than it was in the past. The reason is that the already precarious balance between man and woman has been violently upset of recent years. Formerly one sex was subordinate to the other. This inequality was always a source of sufficiently serious disturbances to make the scales waver, for repression always evokes resistance. Nevertheless, the supremacy of man was so secure, owing to the solidarity of the male sex, that woman had to resign herself to her fate of playing second fiddle. During the last decades, however, as a result of changes in the economic, social and political institutions of human society, masculine supremacy, which had existed since civilization began, was undermined. This gave woman an opportunity for rejecting her subordinate rôle   All men and women individually were then obliged to win a position for themselves in relation to the other sex instead of having their position allotted to them by a hard and fast system.

[129]

THE THREE LIFE TASKS

Woman now seeks to obtain equal rights with man, if she does not strive for superiority as over-compensation for her past subjection Man fears to lose the superiority which was assumed to belong to his sex.

So men and women are now running after a masculine ideal, which no longer corresponds to anything that exists in reality. They measure their own value, expressed in what they are and do, by a standard of masculine superiority, which, as we have seen, they set up for themselves in childhood. This standard can only have corresponded to facts as they were in the time of the absolute autocracy of man. It does not in the least correspond to facts as they are now. Most people have a strong " masculine protest " because their idea of their own value compares so unfavourably with their masculine ideal.

This masculine protest seriously hinders co-operation between sexual partners. Women now revolt much more frequently and violently against the rôle of their sex than they did in the days when they had fewer rights and were kept in greater subjection. Men, too, are troubled more than ever before by doubts as to their own manhood, doubts which sufficiently explain not only their horror of marriage, but also the fear of any deep love relationship which they so frequently betray.

Together with this difficulty in fulfilling the love task, which arises out of the struggle between men and women for prestige, we find the problem of

[130]

LOVE

sexuality. Apparently, however, this second difficulty is quite independent of the first. Very few
people are just as natural in their attitude towards
sexuality as they are towards any other biological
problem of natural science. A very widespread
fear of sexuality weakens the comradeship—already
so deficient—which should exist between man and
woman.

Is there any natural foundation in human modes
of thought and feeling for this special attitude to
sexuality? It is well known that Freud thinks
that the fact of people living together under
civilized conditions, which involves the necessity
for guarding against incest, is responsible. It is at
least true that the human attitude towards
sexuality is characterized by shame. Shame alone
gives certain natural processes a meaning which
they would not otherwise have, and shame is
undoubtedly a product of upbringing. There is
no natural shame. Otherwise the motives for
shame would not differ in different ages and among
different peoples. Shame presupposes the existence of certain laws and rules, the observance of
which it guarantees. The educators try to train
the child to obey the established laws.

The purpose and origin of shame are plainly
recognizable in the view people take of the act of
defecation. The child must learn clean habits if
he is to be properly adjusted to civilized conditions
of life. At first he cannot control his digestive

THE THREE LIFE TASKS

mechanism and naturally at the same time his interest is aroused. The object of upbringing is to change all this. Unfortunately the method generally employed is as unsuitable as most of the methods employed in upbringing. The educators try to suggest to the child that there is something disgusting about metabolic functions and the organs which perform them. This is the method which suggests itself most readily to them since they were familiarized with it through the mistakes of their own upbringing. So they say, " Ugh, how nasty ! How horrible ! No, that isn't at all nice ! You disgusting child ! " The more easily and skilfully the educators can teach the child clean habits, the less emphasis they place on metabolic functions and the more natural the processes of defecation appear.

Children who have ranged themselves against their parents and have some grievance against them are inclined to frustrate the parents' efforts to teach them cleanliness. Educators use terms and expressions of disgust more freely against these children than against any others. It follows that the clean habits which the children do finally learn will be associated in their minds with an unusually keen sense of shame.

Shame is akin to aversion and it is noteworthy that aversion characterizes people who are inclined to resist the laws of the community. Just as shame and aversion indicate that the child is resisting

[132]

LOVE

pressure brought to bear on him by upbringing, these feelings are employed in later life as ready excuses for further evasions of certain tasks.

The close similarity between shame and aversion is the origin of the error which associates defecation with the sexual function and regards a violent desire for defecation as part of the sexual urge. This form of desire is created only when upbringing places a strong emphasis on defecation. Therefore the tendency to regard the excretory organs and the sexual organs with similar feelings of shame and aversion is purely and simply the result of identical educational methods.

The question why do people repudiate their sexual desires by a trick of repression similar to the feeling of shame which distorts their view of the act of defecation now claims our attention. The need for cleanliness certainly complicates the problem of defecation, but why must people subject their sexuality to such a strong external check ?

We know that the Mohammedans, for instance, have particularly strict shame laws. At the same time we are bound to notice that their women have been so shorn of their rights that they have been practically enslaved. Masculine domination has never been so barefaced as it was among the Mohammedans until a short time ago. This is not to be regarded as a coincidence. Subjection of one sex is always found side by side with particularly strict sexual laws, which operate chiefly against the

THE THREE LIFE TASKS

subjected sex. So in the time of the matriarchy men were forced into a position of shame and modesty similar to the position allotted to the women by our social code until the end of the last century.

As people did not know the real reasons, they thought that shame belonged to the nature of woman and attributed its existence to the wisdom of a divine law. Only the collapse of masculine autocracy in our time has made it clear that woman's greater feeling of shame has nothing to do with her function as mother, for even in the time of the matriarchy when shame had not yet taught her to be submissive, she had to bear children. So the sense of shame which society requires of woman proves to be a means for keeping her sexually and personally dependent on man. By demanding virginity and forbidding intercourse outside marriage man kept *virgo intacta* completely in his power.

Shame laws were directed exclusively against woman, but of course they could not fail to impose some checks on man also, even though he showed relatively less shame. First of all, he could not get away from the fact that he always needed a woman as his partner. Secondly, he was obliged to mount guard as husband, father and brother over woman's honour, and lastly he was himself the son of a woman, whose feeling of shame had helped to confuse him when he began to acquire sexual knowledge.

It was necessary to go into this somewhat

[134]

LOVE

lengthy discussion of shame in order to show that even the social problems of sexuality turn entirely on the rivalry between man and woman. Nowadays when the feeling in favour of equality of rights between man and woman is steadily gaining ground, shame complicates sexual problems relatively less, merely because it is no longer necessary for keeping woman in subjection and depriving her of rights. Already it is possible to write and speak openly about these questions. This in itself shows that shame has nothing whatever to do with a danger of incest, which, of course, is hardly more common in our times than it was in the past. Further, this danger does not really exist. Children do not need sexual intercourse with their parents ; neither do healthy parents have such desires. So the fact that human beings live together in civilized communities is not in the least responsible for the tendency to ban sexuality or regulate it by a system of punishments and sanctions.

Nor can any responsibility for this tendency be attached to culture. Culture is not a sublimation of sexuality, but the fulfilment of man's desire to overcome a feeling of weakness and inadequacy.

The nearer we approach the goal of equality of rights between man and woman, and the less danger there is of subjection of one sex to the other, the easier it will become for human beings to regard their sexuality as naturally and fearlessly as any other problem of natural science.

THE THREE LIFE TASKS

Humanity is still under the spell of the fear of everything sexual which has been instilled into every child. Above all, girls can easily get the impression from what they observe and hear and from experiences shared with other people that sexuality involves a special danger for woman. It is a source of disgrace and dishonour. It is the cause of pregnancy with all its perils and suffering. On these grounds a prejudice against men is often formed at an early age. Many women regard themselves as mere objects for satisfying man's needs and think that he derives only pleasure and they only harm from sexuality.

Adolescents will always continue to form mistaken ideas and magnify certain dangers they see in sexuality until explanations of sexuality are made as dispassionate and straightforward as the explanations given in all the other branches of knowledge which help to fit the child for life.

If the educators themselves have no fear of sexuality they need not regard the presentment of sexuality, on which so much depends, as a difficult task. All they have to do is to reply in language which the child can understand to the questions he asks at a very early age—often when he is only three to four years old. If they adhere strictly to the language of the child's questions their explanations will be given naturally and easily, since the child goes on asking questions only in so far as his understanding permits him to frame them.

[136]

LOVE

In addition to the masculine protest (which arises out of the doubt felt by both man and woman in their ability to play a superior masculine rôle) and fear of sexuality, a third difficulty impedes fulfilment of the love task—namely, the difficulty people have in submitting to a union. Anyone who has resented compulsion and dependence in childhood easily imagines that freedom and independence give a secure and lasting feeling of personal value, and anyone who is conscious of being weak fears a close union which may reveal this weakness. As men think they are expected to play a superior rôle but know how little fitted they are to play it well, they fear union much more nowadays than women do. Women on the other hand require the surrender of the man's whole personality, and overestimate the value of such a surrender, because they regard it as a pledge or token which they ought to receive in recognition of the sacrifice they consider they make by yielding. So the sexes turn the question of union into a dispute about prices, each trying to gain an advantage over the other. In particular, the union which involves the most far reaching consequences, that is to say marriage, often proves to be of greater social and economic advantage to the woman than it is to the man. The wish to gain complete possession of somebody is expressed most plainly by jealousy. Jealousy is never a sign of love. It only indicates fear of not being able to hold another person.

THE THREE LIFE TASKS

The rôle of virginity is nowadays complicated by special difficulties connected with sexuality and the real or imaginary sacrifices demanded by union. Although society no longer requires women to practise chastity so strictly as in the past, the transition from virginity to womanhood still represents an insoluble problem for many women. They fear the step which makes them complete women. This is, of course, due both to their upbringing and to their attitude to sexuality. The dread of losing virginity is particularly marked in women who regard everything sexual as beastly and degrading and therefore resent the manifestations of their womanhood, as for example menstruation. (This resentment is the origin of many menstrual and premenstrual disorders.) On the other hand the man no longer regards virginity as an estimable or particularly valuable quality of womanhood. This, of course, is only because he wishes to evade responsibility, because he fears that too close a tie will bind the woman to him, and because—unlike men in the past—he does not want to play the part of the first man in a woman's life. (So he voluntarily surrenders the most characteristic position of masculine supremacy).

In view of what has been said it becomes easy to understand why the love task is seldom satisfactorily fulfilled. It requires the exercise of great courage on the part of each individual. For this reason the love life of so many people is based on

[138]

LOVE

evasion of the real solution, and so many mistaken experiments and evasive arrangements are made by married and unmarried partners.

People betray their want of courage even in their choice of a love partner. We have only to observe how the feeling of love grows and declines to realize over and over again that the human being is not controlled by irresponsible urges, as he likes to think. In reality his intentions control his apparently automatic " urges ". People are easily deceived by an alleged contradiction between emotion and reason. If they cannot justify their intentions by an appeal to reason they say that emotion and reason are irreconcilable and they rely on an emotion, which appears to be independent of their will, and therefore irresponsible, to execute their intentions. Sexuality is by nature without direction. The direction it eventually takes depends entirely on the individual's choice of a personal goal.

Many people drift into unhappy love affairs, chiefly because they are capable of loving only while real union is impossible. They give the impression that they would like to take steps to fulfil the love task. In reality they have no intention of doing so. Instead of admitting that they are at fault in some way, they pretend that they are the victims of their emotions—victims of a fate which stands between them and fulfilment of their desire. Desire and emotion are strongest

THE THREE LIFE TASKS

when the individual is least prepared to take any step in the direction of a real solution. No love seems so passionate as unrequited love, or the love that can never hope for fulfilment because external circumstances make a union impossible. The wildest erotic fancies fill the minds of people who are anxious to evade every practical possibility of a union. In their day dreams they go on a quest which they never undertake in real life. On the other hand their emotion usually begins to decline as soon as it becomes possible for them to realize their "wishes". In this way they show how skilfully they can use their emotion as a weapon for resisting the discipline of a union and for evading reality. Often a love emotion vanishes altogether if the danger of a close union arises. A desire for distance may cause one partner to draw away from the other. This is what happens in marriage when distance, which could be maintained previous to marriage, is inevitably decreased by cohabitation.

A particularly clear example of the way in which emotion can be employed for creating distance is to be found in the tendency to feel an inclination for more than one person at the same time. This is sometimes regarded as an argument in favour of the view that some human beings have dual personalities. The reason why people so often seem to find their physical ideal in one person and their spiritual ideal in another is that they do not

[140]

LOVE

wish to give themselves completely to either, and so are determined to go only halfway in recognizing either. The tendency to create distance in a marriage may be expressed by a sudden passion for a third person. The Don Juan type uses every new love emotion to end an old liaison. It may be that the Don Juan and the vamp owe their numerous conquests to the fact that they are the most unsuitable partners to have.

In particular, all perversions show how people choose wrongly in order to evade the love task. A long training prepares the way for these perversions and accustoms the naturally blind sexual urge to objects which make a natural love choice impossible. Likewise, people who say that they are incapable of experiencing love emotions or allege the impossibility of finding a love partner show that they intend to evade the love task.

Even if a successful love choice is made and leads to marriage or a union outside marriage, the subsequent history of the relationship often shows how perverse the choice really was. It is not at all rare for people to choose and assign a value to their partners chiefly on account of their faults (though, of course, they do not admit this) so that later on they can shift the whole blame for disaster on to the partner. So many people have too little self confidence to try to find lasting happiness in love. They feel all the more uncertain of themselves if in childhood they saw how difficult the love task

[141]

THE THREE LIFE TASKS

could be. It is natural for children whose parents live unhappily together to overestimate the difficulty of this task. In their caution they choose unwisely and give their love to somebody who fulfils their desire for superiority or security. We may be sure that the man who accuses his wife of want of independence chose her for the very reason that her need for someone to lean on made his superiority apparent, and that the man who complains that his wife is masterful and tyrannical really chose that kind of wife because she looked after him, took all responsibility off his shoulders and mothered him.

Under cover of illness also people may attempt to evade a union or to create distance after a union has been consummated. Illness as a mode of evading the love task includes perversions like sexual impotence and frigidity, which are not organic in origin and are therefore forms of neurosis.

Courage to accept a partner of the opposite sex is necessary for fulfilment of the love task. This suggests an answer to the question : What is love ? Desire and acceptance of the partner are identical. If the partners accept each other desire is awakened, and, unless it is intended to keep open a way of retreat, leads to fulfilment of the love task. The partner is not then regarded as a mere object, but is joyfully accepted as a fellow human being. Love is a task for two. When two people completely find each other the problem is solved.

[142]

III

FRIENDSHIP

No one is ever in touch with the whole human community. Each individual is connected with only a few people, but in his relations with them he expresses his attitude to the whole community. Once we know how a man gets on with the other members of his family and his fellow workers, whether he has many friends and how much trouble he takes in order to enjoy the society of other people we have the key to his personality and know more or less what to expect of him. The human being has to establish social relationships and come into contact with other people in order to satisfy an everyday need. The way he behaves to other people is a most trustworthy indication of the quality of his community feeling. If many people whose community feeling is comparatively undeveloped fulfil the occupational task relatively well and if on the other hand people with the average amount of community feeling nowadays encounter special difficulties in fulfilling the love task, each person's social relationships reflect faithfully his attitude to the community. No external pressure compels fulfilment of this task as of the occupational task ; on the other hand,

[143]

THE THREE LIFE TASKS

it is not complicated like the love task by difficulties which go deeper than ordinary human relationships. Everyone is free to decide whether and to what extent he will form friendships, adapt himself to friends and co-operate with them, or whether he will choose solitude and detachment. He uses his judgment spontaneously in these matters. Therefore the way in which he fulfils the task of friendship is the best measure of the strength of his community feeling.[1]

A man who makes a muddle of his social relationships will, of course, try to excuse himself before his own conscience, as he does when he fails in the other life tasks. He will blame the mistakes of others for his own mistaken conduct. He may be inclined to regard all other people as worse than himself—more selfish, more disagreeable, more difficult to get on with. This attitude is adopted by people who are conscious of any kind of deficiency when they compare themselves with others and feel that they cannot quite keep pace with them or compete with them. They can even make a virtue of an inferiority by attributing their failures to their " fineness of feeling ", their good-nature, or some other supposed quality. In the end they withdraw into a "splendid isolation " and seem to think it worth their while to break off their friendships with other people, because the other people deserve nothing better.

[1] Pages 6 and 7.

[144]

FRIENDSHIP

A hostile attitude to the community may be concealed beneath pseudo-ethical or philosophical ideas. It is not at all unusual to find a small clique closing itself against the community. Properly developed community feeling is ready to recognize the needs of a community beyond and above every small group. The small group is generally actuated by selfish interests and tends to range itself against the community just as the neurotic ranges himself against his fellow human beings. Family solidarity frequently helps to strengthen feelings that are hostile to the community. A love union may grow out of the partners' common hostility to other people. It may be a union which seems to offer a complete solution of the love problem, but no attempt is made to solve the problem of wider social relationships. The apparent solidarity of these narrow associations, which are formed from motives of hostility to the great human community, recalls the semblance of solidarity found outside the human community among criminals.

Interest in other people also leads us to make efforts to understand universal problems which unite large groups of people. So the individual's attitude to politics is typical of his attitude to his fellow beings. A man who holds aloof from all political discussions, and does not try to help in any active or positive way to solve the problems of the community, and so does not support any of the existing political movements, betrays his lack of

[145]

THE THREE LIFE TASKS

interest in universal problems. He may excuse himself on the ground that all the political programmes are inadequate and that political life is full of absurdities and abuses. If he were really community minded he would be willing to co-operate even when things are not done just as he thinks they should be done. We never find a community, a movement or a system of thought which entirely corresponds to our views. No one who is continually emphasizing how much he differs from other people and regards the differences as all-important will be able to co-operate. The individualist arrives at his intellectual and emotional conclusions by a private logic, which is biased by secret hostility to other people and amounts to hostility to the whole community.

Reserved feelings may be concealed by exaggerations in social relationships just as easily as by any other tricks. Many people who are very active in politics and other spheres are actuated less by social interest than by will-to-power, and many ultra-sociable people are secretly lonely and isolated. Even the hail-fellow-well-met person can make it impossible for other people to get any idea of what he is really like by keeping his inmost thoughts, feelings, conflicts and problems to himself. He takes refuge in sociability in order to evade more significant human relationships, whether in his family or in a circle of friends.

[146]

EPILOGUE

ANYONE who has grasped the simple truths upon which Individual Psychology has been built up soon realizes why people under-rate it and why acceptance of it involves certain difficulties. It provides a set of very simple tools for investigating complex character formations. Simplicity characterizes the fundamental laws of community feeling, its counterpart the inferiority feeling (which is the source of all striving for significance), the unity of the personality and the individual life style. Whoever refuses to allow himself to be convinced that such laws govern all the activities of the mind forgets that fundamental laws have always proved to be simple in essence though applicable to complex modes of life. One has only to think of Newton's law of gravitation, which enabled so many varieties of motion of inanimate matter to be deduced from the same fundamental formula. It is not surprising, therefore, that it should be possible to apply the fundamental laws discovered by Alfred Adler to *all* psychological manifestations. How little justification there is in the accusation that these laws fail to take equipment and the part played by the instincts into account is shown in the chapters this book devotes to those subjects.

EPILOGUE

All these objections have a deeper significance. It is evident that the teachings of Individual Psychology are intelligible to all, and many people even agree with them so long as no personal problem appears to be attacked. The findings of Individual Psychology win their assent when they refer to other people, but they try to feel sceptical and raise objections as soon as their own behaviour comes under observation. They object that our laws cannot explain everything. Yet it is significant that each one takes exception to something different while readily assenting to statements which another person has difficulty in accepting. Whoever has deeply explored human nature will have no difficulty in understanding this. Everyone refuses to understand what does not agree with his life plan and involves the recognition of his own responsibility. This explains why people are constantly emphasizing the special importance of the equipment and the instincts. They represent the greatest limitation of individual responsibility.

Our critics behave like our patients. Patients assent without much difficulty while the laws of individual conduct are being stated in a general way. But the moment any scientific statement seems likely to have a personal application their understanding halts. And when they are no longer able to deny the logic of our arguments they try as a last resource to explain their standpoint by saying : " *Practically* everything you say is true,

EPILOGUE

but all the same there must be something else which ought to be taken into account." This attitude may be observed in patients even after an undeniable cure with cessation of the symptoms has been wrought. The five per cent which these patients regard as excepted from the laws of Individual Psychology is intended to enable them to fall back on the old excuses of illness and inability, etc., whenever in a new set of difficulties they see a favourable opportunity for doing so. Only exposure of this fraud makes it possible to destroy the fiction of a residuum which has nothing to do with personal responsibility.

Thus both in general discussions and in psychotherapeutical treatment Individual Psychology arouses the most violent resistance the moment it establishes as a fact the responsibility of the individual. The knowledge it gives is not so comforting as other teachings, which maintain that the character of the individual is determined by such factors as heredity, organic changes occurring in the nervous system, the development of instincts, external circumstances, environment and economic and social burdens. Anyone who tries to excuse himself is always finding fresh opportunities for doing so, and in order to refute the unwelcome statements of Individual Psychology he can always refer to contrary systems of thought. Who can tell which system is right ?

The question of objective knowledge represents

[149]

EPILOGUE

an extraordinarily difficult and complicated problem of metaphysics. Apparently there is no such thing as an absolute truth. It seems that reason originated as a weapon which was employed by man in his struggle for existence—in his endeavour to overcome his natural weakness. So each human being still employs reason as a weapon and recognizes it only as it helps him to reach the goal at which he is aiming. Faced with two scientifically established psychological principles which flatly contradict each other, no one can determine with certainty how much truth and how much error one of them contains. We reach our decisions subjectively, or a chance opportunity may help us to become more closely acquainted with a certain idea, or we decide in favour of an opinion because it agrees with our own views—which are determined by our own problems.

So we know what to expect when we have to treat a patient who has undergone a previous course of treatment based on another system of psycho-therapy. Such a patient may welcome the teachings of Individual Psychology. They are new to him and explain much that formerly seemed unintelligible. But sooner or later comes the moment when the patient resists. May not our way of looking at things be wrong, seeing that so-and-so maintains something quite different ? Experience shows that this attitude merely indicates that we have now touched upon a problem

[150]

EPILOGUE

which the patient is unwilling should be discovered. This resistance, which Psycho-Analysis also describes when discussing treatment, is roused not by the detection of sexual problems, but by the patient's unwillingness to recognize his own responsibility. Because he does not wish to confess what his goal really is, he refuses to have anything to do with knowledge which might explain what it is and why he chose it. " Private sense " resists common sense.

Of course, the significance underlying the patient's resistance does not entitle a psycho-therapist to assert whatever seems right to him and to think that every objection to his assertions proves that they are correct. Contested views are not proved to be correct merely by the fact of their being contested. But impartial and expert examination of the situation described above shows that the patient's resistance is always an expression of fear—fear of having to recognize his own responsibility, of having to make a decision, of having to give up safeguards.

It is not for us as Individual Psychologists to argue whether we are right or not. Anyone who examines our findings with an open and impartial mind will hardly be able to escape their logic and will find them confirmed at every point in everyday life. It would be useless for us to go into the question of metaphysical proofs and hypotheses. Such discussions have little to do with practical

[151]

EPILOGUE

life. The only thing we can do, whether we have to deal with patients, teachers or any of our fellow beings, is to appeal to the reason, common sense and conscience of all. We know that the most advanced minds are working along the same lines as Individual Psychology, and we share with all advanced thinkers the desire to help the race to found a real community of all human beings, which will recognize instead of upper and lower classes only fellow beings and fellow workers.